PRAISE FOR
GET GROUNDED, GET WELL

"Dr. Sinatra has been one of my go-to experts, teachers, and good luck charms for his insights and advice on keeping the body healthy. When he first explained grounding to me, I incorporated it into my own life and really noticed the difference, especially in the quality of my sleep. But after experiencing a bad fall, I found that grounding was not only a big part of my recovery—it was lifesaving."

> —Suzanne Somers, actress and author of *TOX-SICK*
> *and A New Way to Age*

"A clear, well-researched, essential guide to wellness and natural healing. Highly recommended!

> —Michael J. Gelb, author of *How to Think Like*
> *Leonardo Da Vinci*

"*Get Grounded, Get Well* elegantly lays out the science and practical application behind the most important health discovery of the millennium—grounding. Cowritten by America's beloved integrative cardiologist Dr. Stephen Sinatra, his very knowledgeable son Step, and passionate grounding advocate, Sharon Whiteley, this book will not only save your life, but save humanity from the chronic ailments of modern society."

> —Ann Louise Gittleman, PhD, CNS, multiple
> award-winning nutritionist and *New York Times*
> bestselling author of more than thirty-six books

GET GROUNDED, GET WELL

GET

Connect to the Earth

GROUNDED

to Improve Your Health,

GET

Well-Being, and Energy

WELL

STEPHEN SINATRA, MD,
SHARON WHITELEY,
AND STEP SINATRA

FOREWORD BY DAVE ASPREY

HAMPTON ROADS

Cover design by Sky Peck Design
Interior by Happenstance Type-O-Rama
Typeset in Goudy and Avenir

Hampton Roads Publishing Company, Inc.
Charlottesville, VA 22906
Distributed by Red Wheel/Weiser, LLC
www.redwheelweiser.com

Sign up for our newsletter and special offers by going to www.redwheelweiser.com
/newsletter.

ISBN: 978-1-64297-048-7

Library of Congress Cataloging-in-Publication Data

Names: Sinatra, Stephen T., author. | Whiteley, Sharon, author. | Sinatra,
    Step, author.
Title: Get grounded, get well : connect to the Earth to improve your
    health, well-being, and energy / Stephen T. Sinatra, Sharon Whiteley,
    and Step Sinatra.
Description: Charlottesville, VA : Hampton Roads, [2023] | Summary: "Nature
    has been the world's most acclaimed healer since the beginning of time,
    with time-tested references to its ability to heal body, mind, and soul,
    dating to the earliest civilizations. This book offers readers the
    secret to better health through grounding. Grounding, the simple act of
    connecting to the always-abundant, nourishing energy of the Earth's
    surface, has been scientifically and medically proven through numerous
    studies to have significant positive effects on our physiology. It helps
    to restore energy, improve circulation, alleviate stress, help ensure a
    better night's sleep, reduce inflammation, and much more"—Provided by
    publisher.
Identifiers: LCCN 2022051089 | ISBN 9781642970487 (paperback) | ISBN
    9781612834870 (kindle edition)
Subjects: LCSH: Energy medicine—Popular works. | Nature, Healing power
    of—Popular works. | Magnetic healing—Popular works. | Electromagnetism
    in medicine. | BISAC: HEALTH & FITNESS / Alternative Therapies | HEALTH
    & FITNESS / Diet & Nutrition / General
Classification: LCC RZ421 .S56 2023 | DDC 615.8/52—dc23/eng/20221214
LC record available at https://lccn.loc.gov/2022051089

Printed in the United States of America
IBI
10 9 8 7 6 5 4 3 2 1

A Word from the Authors

Having access to health information empowers us to make important decisions regarding our own well-being. Given the wealth of medical information that is available online, in the news, in scientific journals, and through other sources, it can be both overwhelming and confusing to ascertain which protocol to follow. Health information is constantly changing as a result of new research and various approaches to treating different conditions. So it's hard to know which is the best advice for you.

As healing advocates, we have made it our mission to share what we know about modalities that work in your best interests. We know that we can improve our health by changing our habits and lifestyles, including eating organic foods, exercising every day, and avoiding harmful toxins in our diet and environment. In many cases, we can even reverse diseases naturally, without turning to prescribed medicines. People who have discovered the secret sauce to a healthier life have added grounding to their daily routine, like the residents of Earth's "Blue Zones" who live to be a hundred years or older in good health. We believe that grounding is a big reason why they live so long.

In fact, we believe that grounding is the antidote for millions of people. It's also one of the greatest kept secrets when it comes to our health. Only a small part of the population knows about this. Once people realize that grounding is free, and it is healing, especially in this enormous inflammatory time we live in, it will have an incredible effect on public health. The breadth of validation from trustworthy data and real-life testimonials is absolutely enormous.

As Hippocrates said, "Nature is the best medicine." And with centuries-long evidence to support that heralded dogma, that is one piece of medical wisdom that you can count on.

—STEPHEN SINATRA, MD, SHARON WHITELEY, AND STEP SINATRA

Contents

Foreword

When I was in the process of starting the biohacking movement a dozen years ago, I admit I was a little reluctant to include grounding, also known as Earthing.

But I did it anyway. Here's why. Early in my career, I had the exhausting responsibility of flying from California to Cambridge, England, every single month and spending a week there. It was jet lag hell.

I decided to try everything under the sun that might possibly help me adapt more quickly to such a brutal travel regimen. I landed on the idea that exercise after I landed would raise my body temperature and tell my body that it was morning.

The first time I tried it, it was the rare sunny day in London, so I did yoga in the park. I felt amazing. No jet lag. No sore joints. My brain worked just fine. I had solved the problem!

The next trip, there was the stereotypical London fog, so I exercised indoors. On carpet. My brain was fuzzy. My joints were sore. The jet lag was worse than ever. My experiment had failed.

It was only after coming across Dr. Sinatra's amazing body of research that I had my personal eureka moment. It wasn't the exercise. It was being barefoot in the park doing yoga. It wasn't the yoga. It was the Earth.

It takes a rare and curious mind to notice something that makes a difference for your health and performance when that thing is so common and unexpected that you could easily miss it.

I am now 100 percent convinced that electrical activity in our bodies is responsible for how we age, how we feel, how we think, and even how we treat other people.

And what could be more fundamental to electrical activity than having a high-quality grounding experience? Anyone who has studied engineering the way I did before I became a biohacker understands that current doesn't flow without a good ground.

Dr. Sinatra, one of the co-authors, along with grounding experts, Sharon Whiteley and Step Sinatra, states emphatically in the excellent book you are about to read that "grounding is one of the most important health discoveries of the last 50 years." I heartily agree with his assessment.

You aren't going to see hundred-million-dollar double-blind placebo-controlled trials of grounding paid for by pharmaceutical companies anytime soon. That's because everything is free. It's powerful. It can help you lower your stress, have more energy, clear up your brain, reduce chronic pain, and just feel connected to the world.

I invite you to absorb every single word in this precious book. And do it barefoot. On the Earth. 🙏

—DAVE ASPREY

INTRODUCTION
The World's First
Healing Resource

You may not be familiar with the term *grounding*, but it has been around since the beginning of time, making it the very first healing resource in the world. It came into being the moment life began on Earth, some 3.5 billion years ago, providing an energetic connection between the planet and the life it sustains simply by shared contact. Nature as healer came next, providing every living being with the nourishment and nutrition they needed to survive and thrive. The human body itself is another powerful healing force, housing the most sophisticated self-contained health systems ever created so we can self-heal under the right conditions.

For a long time, these three health resources were all we needed to stay well.

The Earth's surface keeps our bodies in balance through a constant exchange of electrons and electric vibrations that literally recharge us with positive healing energy. That's the essence of grounding, and you can do it while you are out walking, swimming, gardening, or doing anything that puts you in direct contact with the Earth. Until the end of the 19th century, grounding was a seamless part of everyday life. People walked everywhere either barefoot or in pure leather footwear, along dirt and stone surfaces, each of which is naturally conductive to Earth's energy flow, unknowingly grounding as they went and keeping a host of opportunistic illnesses at bay. Interestingly, inflammation, the bane of modern-day health, was unheard of back then. Diabetes was unknown. People didn't typically die from heart disease, hypertension, and any number of chronic conditions that confound doctors today. They didn't commonly exist when grounding was in the mix, or if they did, they were rather infrequent events.

Back in the days before agribusiness was big business, nature made all our food, organically and sustainably. Pesticides and toxic chemical fertilizers were nonexistent. Genetically modified foods were the stuff of science fiction. Fish was fresh caught from seas devoid of pollution, heavy metals, and plastics. Meats weren't processed or injection fed. We literally lived on the land, growing what we had, harvesting what we could.

Earth was our lifeline. Nature was our lifeblood. And our bodies and our health were sustained by them.

But modern-day technologies and lifestyles have changed all that.

We live in a world that is increasingly man made and disconnected from the life-giving properties of the Earth. From synthetic footwear and nonconductive building materials and road surfaces that prevent us from grounding, to toxic water, processed foods, and environmental pollutants that impact our food sources, to disruptive electromagnetic field and electromagnetic computer, Wi-Fi, and cellular waves that trigger allergens and viruses, today's world has changed our health, and not in good ways.

We suffer from debilitating ailments that weaken our immune systems and rob us of our energy. We tire easily, hurt more, sleep less, ache a lot, heal slowly, stress out, and suffer from heart-related, diabetic, and autoimmune issues that become more serious by the day. Inflammation is at the heart of the diseases we are seeing today, and left unchecked, the end results are devastating.

How do we live in this toxic environment of not only plastics and petrochemicals, heavy metals, and air pollution, but also with inflammatory diseases and infectious viruses like Lyme disease and COVID-19 and its variants? How can mankind adapt? And why haven't we heard more about grounding?

You'll find the answers—and the antidote—in this book.

As a doctor, entrepreneur, and healer, each of the three of us discusses the big, simple, heal-for-free aspects of grounding as a solution to modern man's enigma of living in the world today. We'll take you from ancient lands to hallowed grounds, inside cities and outside in parks, tracing the path of grounding through the ages to present day. We'll tell you where you can ground and where you shouldn't. We'll explain what to do and when, why grounding is important, and how it can literally save your life.

You'll hear our own personal stories, from Sharon's life-altering bout with a sudden heart attack to Step's deathbed survival to Stephen's life-changing lifestyle where grounding is incorporated into every step he takes on his journey to stay well.

We'll back them up with science, clinical studies, and statistics, sharing research and findings, easy to understand and hard to dismiss. We'll show you how grounding has helped heal others—and how it can help you stay healthy for the long run.

Our motivation for writing this book is simple and straightforward. We walk the talk and believe without a doubt that grounding is one of greatest health discoveries ever. We hope you'll want to pass the torch and spread the word so that others may benefit from grounding, too.

Why isn't it front-page news? It should be. It has helped people survive everything from coronary events to COVID-19, and it will continue to work wonders as viruses and vascular issues become more prevalent in the future.

Grounding, like nature, is simple and subtle, and some people just don't get it. It doesn't come in a pill or a bottle. You don't need a prescription or a doctor to benefit from it. You can get grounded everywhere at every age and any time. You can do it indoors and out, while you are sleeping and when you're awake. You can't overdo it or become over grounded. It's endless, abundant, and always free. And it's the best way to do great things for your body.

Are you ready to get grounded and get well?

1

THE GREATEST HEALTH DISCOVERY ON EARTH

Storytelling is information sharing at its best. It pairs faces with facts, experiences with expertise, and recommendations with references personally tested. The stories and testimonies you will read in this book about the healing benefits of grounding are all compelling evidence about a health resource that has been available to all of us since we first walked on Earth. As co-authors whose grounding practices changed our lives—and, in the case of two of us, actually saved our lives—we have become passionate advocates of grounding as a way of life. We've done the research, analyzed the studies, and made the connections, standing steadfastly by our beliefs and convictions that Mother Nature really does know best when it comes to our well-being.

In other words, we crossed all the "t's" and dotted all the "i's" before we got together to write this book. As a doctor with five decades of experience as a cardiologist and a psychotherapist, Dr. Sinatra believes in integrative medicine, approaching it from a holistic point of view. "I have made it my mission to explore all the options available to people in their quest for better health. Sure, I believe in proven medical techniques and surgical interventions. They work. But there are other non-invasive preventative ways to help keep a person healthy as well. Nutrition and diet are key, of course. Exercise is a given, as is a good night's sleep. These are no brainers. While people today embrace these commonly accepted practices, grounding, one of the easiest ways to keep your body healthy, has not received the mainstream attention it should."

Until now.

Truth be told, we've encountered a fair number of naysayers along the way who adamantly dismiss the idea that something as simple as a walk in the park can make a difference in how you feel. But it does. And we'll tell you why.

When we began writing this book, the world was in quarantine. As the news of a killer virus spread to every country around the globe, people hunkered down inside their homes, away from crowds and the dreaded COVID-19. Being cooped up caused a cascade of wellness issues, from depression and despondency to weight gain and more. Many postponed medical visits, ignored unsettling symptoms, and feared opening their doors to the outside.

As the months dragged on, medical experts, seeing an onslaught of quarantine-related health issues from our increasingly sedentary and solitary lifestyles, suggested we go back to nature, the exact place we need the most, to start feeling good again. Even with masks on, that "medical advice" helped many of us regain our footing on the path to better health as we took to the trails and the ocean shores, keeping socially distant and staying away from crowded places.

As more and more people began to rediscover our parklands, beaches, lakes, forested playgrounds, and even their own backyards, they also experienced the greatest health discovery on Earth, grounding. They just didn't know it.

The escalating inflammatory diseases and immune deficiencies we are seeing in people today add urgency to our quest to help you get grounded. They include autoimmune diseases, heart disease, high blood pressure, diabetes, and even rogue viruses that send us scurrying indoors for more than a year. Many are exacerbated by our disconnection from the Earth. We believe it's time everyone knows what we are up against in our world today. We want you to be aware of what's good for you—and what's not. The more knowledge you have about grounding, the more empowered you'll become with regard to your own health.

Before we get into the science and the studies that back up the benefits of grounding, we want you to hear our own unscripted stories—how we first heard of grounding, what made us believers, how it helped us, how it connected us, and how we live today, in the hopes you'll discover common ground in them.

They start here.

✿

My name is Sharon Whiteley. I am a serial entrepreneur, retail innovator, and co-author of this book. I've built and sold businesses, invented and marketed products to make people's lives easier and enhance their well-being, written books, and mentored many on their quest for creating innovative merchandise and following their dreams. I created motivational messages for paper products and soft goods, creating the category for milestone occasions and positive aging, pioneered the creation of pop-up and vendor pushcarts for transitory merchandising, unearthed silver gems that kill germs, and was the first to design and produce grounding shoes that help heal you. But of all the experiences and expertise I have shared throughout my life, the stories you will read in the following pages about the life-saving benefits of grounding are among the most meaningful of all.

Have you ever thought that connecting with someone out of the blue, someone who would change your life, was not just a mere coincidence? That your chance meeting was not happenstance, after all? That the spontaneous turn you took, the random book you picked up, or the unplanned, spur-of-the-moment lecture you curiously sauntered into was all part of the universe's grand plan to give you what you need at the moment you needed it?

I hadn't until a chain of synchronistic events, life-altering ones as they turned out to be, made me reconsider the possibilities of things I had never before considered.

It was during the December holidays, over a decade ago, when my friend Carolyn Chin called to see if I was interested in going to a positive aging conference with her, in Las Vegas no less. I was free and didn't have any other plans that day, so I said, sure, what the heck. I could use a little advice on how to survive and grow older gracefully.

The conference was a mecca for anyone interested in the latest advances in integrative healthcare and the newest, most innovative protocols and practices. The exhibit hall was packed with anti-aging remedies, everything from supplements to high-tech freeze-yourself-to-last-forever products. High-profile medical professionals and keynote speakers were sharing their knowledge in a head-turning roster of presentations that, even at this very early hour, were filling fast. But it was a lecture by Dr. Stephen Sinatra that caught my eye that day. I made my way through the cigarette smoke that was already wafting in the air, past the clinks and ka-chings of thirsty slot machines whirring promises of easy money, into the room where the doctor had already begun to speak.

The first thing I heard Dr. Sinatra say, after he introduced himself as a cardiologist with four decades of experience under his belt, was that heart disease was the number one killer of women. Little did I know that it was a foreshadowing comment that would reconnect us some thirteen years later.

He then went on to talk about nature-deficient disorder and how children were being deprived of all the natural health-giving benefits they can access outside. Interesting, I thought as I heard him segue to a topic I also knew nothing about, Earthing and grounding. I had never heard of Earthing before and I thought grounding was something you did to kids when they blew curfew.

What he said was intriguing and solid and I wanted to hear more. He talked about the Earth's energy field and the electrons it released. And I got it. Thank goodness I had paid attention in science class all those years ago when I learned about its electrically charged surface. Dr. Sinatra spoke about how the Earth gives off nourishing energy known as electrons. He explained that our bodies are also electrical systems that benefit from those electrons. When people first populated our planet, he explained in his easy, grounded way, they went barefoot. They connected their bodies, skin to soil, directly to the Earth's surface naturally, day and night. When they first used foot coverings to protect their feet from the cold or the cuts from rough terrain, they made them from pure leather skins. Leather hides and some metals are naturally conductive, which means they allow for the transfer of the electrons between the Earth and living bodies. Our ancestors didn't have many of the chronic illnesses we see today. When footwear went synthetic, and the ground we walk upon was paved over with nonconductive materials, people's health began to suffer in a big way. As we disconnected from Earth, incidences of diabetes, heart disease, high blood pressure, and more skyrocketed. Grounding, the simple act of reconnecting with Earth's energy, said Dr. Sinatra, was the best way to bring those out-of-control modern-day afflictions back down to Earth and give us back our health. And it was free! I was hooked. Who wouldn't be?

After his lecture, I walked around the Exhibit Hall amidst hundreds of booths with this new health discovery setting up shop in my head. Before I knew it, I was standing in front of a booth that was selling Earthing products, and I literally bought everything they had. I didn't know how they worked, but I intuitively knew that they would change my life. Fifteen feet down the aisle, I stopped in my tracks and said, Shoes! What better way to get grounded than through your feet.

As I was flying back to New York City through Tucson, Arizona, to visit a friend, my satchel bulging with purchases that would let me plug into the Earth when I was inside, I couldn't stop thinking about what Dr. Sinatra had said about the healing effects of grounding. Excited, I called another friend of mine when I landed in Arizona—Dr. Ann Marie Chiasson, who was an allopathic family medicine physician, an integrative medicine doc, and an energy medicine practitioner among other health-oriented pursuits—to tell her about my discovery of this new thing called grounding. I can picture her rolling her eyes as she said, "Geez Sharon, you're a nature person, you're smart and interested in all this natural stuff. How is it that you have never heard about grounding?"

That conversation led to important synchronistic introductions to people in the forefront of grounding research—first to Dr. Melinda H. Conner, D.D., Ph.D., AMP, FAM, energy researcher, professor, and author, who immediately encouraged me to locate and talk to one of the country's leading biophysicists, energy medicine expert, acclaimed author, and leading pioneer behind grounding, Jim Oschman in New Hampshire. I got on a plane the next day during a snowstorm to meet Jim and Nora Oschman. Six months later he introduced me to Clint Ober, the man credited with actually rediscovering Earthing itself and how to get the Earth's revitalizing electrons into one's body while indoors through products that plugged into grounding ports. And wouldn't you know it, they were all close associates of Dr. Sinatra, along with many other scientific research collaborators.

Had I not ventured into his lecture so many years ago, I would probably never have known about grounding, let alone devoted the last seventeen years of my life to it. Since then I have founded two shoe companies, Pluggz footwear and Harmony 783, to design and manufacture specially crafted, proprietary grounding shoes; co-written a book about grounding with Dr. Chiasson called *Barefoot Wisdom: Better Health Through Grounding* with a foreword written by Dr. Sinatra himself; healed my life-long bout with Raynaud's disease; and lived to tell the story of emergency room doctors asking me if I had a living will because I had just ninety minutes left to live when I was delivered there by a fire truck ambulance and told I was having a heart attack.

I have been a physician for fifty years, and the two greatest decisions I have ever made in my lifetime have been the utilization of Coenzyme Q10 in my practice, as well as the utilization of Earthing and grounding. Both are powerful electron donors that can help heal a person. Ongoing research continues to shed new light on their ability to combat many modern-day diseases, and we discover something new about them every day. I graduated from medical school in May of 1972, proudly becoming Dr. Sinatra a half a century ago. One of the things about being a doctor is that you never stop learning. You learn from patients you treat, professors you study with, fellow doctors you work with, and very gifted individuals you happen to come across, either in a book, at a lecture, or just by a freak occurrence.

There was a book I read years ago that had a big impact on me and still resonates with me today. It was called *Vibrational Medicine* by Dr. Richard Gerber and it came out in 1987. I was already a doctor by that time, and I remember reading it and realizing that this doctor was decades ahead of his time. I mean decades ahead. He talked about Lyme disease in the book, but he didn't call it Lyme disease. He mentioned that there were going to be parasitic-type of illnesses coming out that mankind needed to face, and it was absolutely amazing. I wondered how a doctor in his thirties could write a book like this. A doctor myself, I thought it was impossible. So I started asking questions and looking for answers from some of my intuitive "spiritual healer" friends. I asked them if they knew of Dr. Gerber. What they relayed to me was that his book was downloaded from spirit. They believed, as I did, that he had channeled the information from some higher source because one human being could not possibly write a book this complicated and thorough. It would take somebody with a PhD, MD, and DDS to really understand the things he writes about. You've got to be prepped for this book, and I read and reread it several times, knowing that he was on to something. The biggest takeaway for me was his assertion that vibrational energy is key to life, key to illness, and the key to being well. I knew it was *the* key; there was no doubt about it.

So when Clint called me some twenty years ago and asked me to join him at an American College of Cardiology meeting to talk about grounding and Earthing, I was prepared. I was so prepped by who I was and where I was lecturing, by reading Gerber's book and by being privy to W. Brugh Joy's transformational work on the potentials for healing with body energies, which, by the way, Sharon also knows about and believes in after years of studying with Brugh Joy himself, that I didn't hesitate. A lot of scientists and doctors who met Clint thought he was crazy. I thought he was a genius.

When Clint presented his ideas and the concept of grounding to me, I loved it. I thought it made sense and I wanted to help him get the word out. I told him that he needed to validate his discovery with clinical studies. He needed to have them published in medical publications even though he would face endless rejections and spend millions of dollars doing it.

I was already familiar with the process from my experience with Coenzyme Q 10. I told him grounding was going to need decades of introspection by professors, PhDs, and naysayers. There were going to be people who believed in it and people who didn't. And there would be controversy, lots of it, with science versus not-science dissertations.

I was used to it. Clint wasn't. But with all the warnings and advice I dispensed, he stayed the course. This book is testament to his findings and the future of a discovery that could very possibly win the Nobel Prize in the upcoming years when people finally understand how incredible it is.

You'll discover why as you get into the real-life information and personal experiences we share with you here. They include my own journey with grounding and how it has become the essence of life and health for me now. You'll also follow Sharon's story, and my son Step's valiant battle back from death's door through grounding.

Like Sharon and me, Step has dedicated his life to grounding, especially after defying a diagnosis that gave him a 1 percent chance of survival. A Wall Street warrior, he had inexplicably wasted away to 87 pounds from a robust 200. He was trying to heal himself, but it was obvious to anyone who saw him during that terrible time that he was dying.

As a last resort, he had traveled to Palm Beach for treatment, but nothing was working. He called us, asking for help, seeking comfort and support. When his mother and I arrived, he was so dehydrated that he needed to have a catheter inserted inside his heart to give him the nutrition his body needed to survive. His surgeon struggled in vain to get a catheter in his shrunken vein. Defeated, he turned to me, knowing that I had done this procedure hundreds of times, and asked, "Can you put a pair of gloves on?" At that moment, I was no longer Step's father, I was his doctor. My son was now my patient and a very sick one at that. Could I pull this off, I wondered?

I did, rejoicing in a short-lived victory that was disrupted by his doctor's sobering words. "We've got to pull a rabbit out of the hat here. Your son needs something way above what we can do for him here."

I was fortunate to know someone with a private jet, and I did not hesitate to call in a favor. Could he fly us back to Connecticut where Step could see a specialist who might be able to save him? Right now?

The doctor was renowned for his work with hyperalimentation, or parenteral nutrition (TPN) as it is commonly known, for premature babies who can't eat. He had groundbreaking success with premature beagle puppies and pioneered the life-saving treatment for critically ill children.[1] Would he be able to do the same for Step? We boarded the plane for what seemed like an arduously long three-hour flight before that question could be answered.

We met him at Waterbury Hospital at one o'clock in the morning where he assessed my son's condition on the spot. He didn't mince his words as he spoke to Step.

"You have a 1 percent chance of making it."

Like Sharon, he made it against all odds.

We later found out that Step was suffering from the perfect storm of metabolic, endocrine, and immune diseases related to toxic EMF exposure. If you have multisystemic illnesses—neurological, endocrinological, and immunological all at the same time—and crazy symptoms like trouble sleeping, digestive problems, sore throats, and more that just keep on presenting, I can tell you from my years of experience that you may be suffering from undiagnosed Lyme disease, chronic black mold exposure, or toxic vibrations that you can't see, taste, or feel, but that will make you very sick, or all three. That's what happened in Step's case, and he'll tell you more in his story. Basically, grounding helped him get his life back, which is why he's so committed to it.

You'll hear the details in the following chapters. They are the reason why each of us has incorporated grounding into our lives, not just now and then or half-heartedly when we think of it, but full on, every day, whether we are inside or out.

We know what grounding can do for you, and it doesn't take much effort on your part. Take the time to step outside and catch some good vibrations from the Earth every day. How much time is enough? Thirty minutes a day is a great start. The point is to make your interactions with the Earth a part of your normal lifestyle.

Dr. Sinatra has put five decades of medicine into this book to give you expert insights on the greatest discoveries he has ever made in his lifetime. Sharon Whiteley has created seven companies all focused on positivity and enhancing people's well-being with seventeen years in this arena. Step Sinatra has made it his mission to help others get grounded. It goes without saying that we need to find ways to detox from the dangers of modern-day living now more than ever. We live in a soup of EMF, computers, Wi-Fi, cordless and cellular phones, and this electromagnetic energy is destroying our DNA. We live in a sea of chemicals and genetically modified organism (GMO) foods. The world's population is at risk, not only from killer viruses but also killer environments.

We are going to tell you how to protect yourself, how to get back to nature, how to get back to grounding, and how to get back to basics. We will show you how to do the things that make sense, that don't cost you anything, that aren't going to hurt you. We'll share the good, the bad, and the ugly with you, too, giving you caveats you need to know so you can make sound decisions for yourself. What we are giving you here is life-saving, it's a gift. And it begins the instant you connect to the Earth.

Read on and find out how to protect your own body, how to be your own detective, your own doctor, your own healer. One of the pearls of this book is to enlighten you about healing your own body and staying well. And as you'll learn, grounding is not only a very simple way to do it, it's one of the most important health discoveries you'll ever make.

2

SACRED GROUND

The Earth has the ability to transform lives. The raw physical beauty of its landscapes automatically recalibrate your sense of wonder as they recharge and restore your energy. Touch it and more miraculous things happen, healing body, mind, and soul with an abundance of natural resources as old as time itself.

The ancients knew about Earth's powers long before science did, of course, naturally benefitting from its nourishment by their simple lifestyles alone. They lived as one with the Earth, sleeping on the ground, bathing in its oceans, rivers, lakes, and streams, walking barefoot or clad in animal-hide shoes, and hand-planting and handpicking herbs, vegetables, and fruits directly from their soil-rooted sources.

Early humans lived according to nature's calendar, going about their daily lives in synchronicity with the intrinsic rhythms of the Earth. They woke at dawn and slept when it was dark, instinctively staying in concert with the circadian rhythm that occurs as the Earth turns on its axis on any given day. They tuned into the seasonal rhythm of the Earth by necessity, taking their cues from the Earth's orbit around the sun, staying warm and gathering food in summer, storing provisions and seeking shelter in caves and huts during the cold winter months. Each activity kept them in direct contact with the Earth, nourishing them with the natural energy that was always underfoot 24/7. They spent their days grounding, although they didn't know it at the time.

Almost every living organism has an internal biological clock that synchronizes its behavior with the environment in which it lives. Endogenous biological clocks follow the solar-influenced 24-hour transition of day and night, the tidal 12.4 hour rising and falling of the tides that is governed by the lunar cycle, and the annual seasonal changes.

The tidal rhythm, the gravitational ebb and flow of the oceans, corresponds with our body's own oceans inside; we are, after all, composed of 55 (women) to 60 (men) percent water, making us susceptible to the pull of the sun and the moon.

Dr. Sinatra met a woman who described herself as a bush Indian not too long ago at a rustic beach bar in the Bahamas. "I had just come in from fly fishing in a slack tide and the fish were hitting. My bare feet were covered in sand and the rest of me was dripping wet from wading in the surf. There were a few people sitting at the bar and the TV was on overhead, the channel turned to, of all things, the *Dr. Oz* show. I happened to be on that episode, discussing the *Great Cholesterol Myth* with Mehmet Oz and Dr. Jonny Bowden. Frankly, I thought to myself as I looked around at my fellow patrons, this isn't their thing and no one will notice me. But then I saw the bartender looking at me, then looking back up at the screen. With my newly grown beard and casual beachcomber attire, I hardly resembled my TV persona, but she recognized me and immediately started up a conversation.

As luck would have it, she was a healer, a woman who had grown up learning about natural healing techniques that were passed down from her ancestors through the generations. We started talking about herbal medicine and holistic healing modalities, and it led to stories about how she used the outgoing tide as a way of healing the body. Taking stock of my wet appearance, she said, "when you are standing in the waves on the seashore, gravity brings the blood down to your feet. The ebbing tide pulls against the body and discharges toxins through your feet, cleansing the body of harmful elements naturally."

Coincidentally, I had just finished reviewing a book written by cardiovascular surgeon Dr. Gerry Lamole, Dr. Oz's father-in-law, about keeping the lymph system healthy. The lymphatic system serves as our body's maintenance department, harvesting toxins taken from the bloodstream and internal organs, and it has a direct effect on our cardiovascular, neurological, and immune systems. If we keep the lymph flow going, it can help eliminate toxins from our body.

How can we do that? One of the best ways of keeping the flow moving, believe it or not, is to bounce around on a trampoline, discharging the sludge physically. You can also go to a sauna and sweat out these impurities, which is what Native Americans have done for hundreds of years in sweat lodges. A lot of the toxins that harm your body lie just beneath the surface of the skin, including mercury, insecticides, and pesticides, and are easily released from the body through sweating. There are also herbal remedies you can use to help move lymph flow as well as certain maneuvers you can do, including the up and down arm movements employed by conductors during orchestral performances. Interestingly there are more classical music conductors who lived to be over 100 years old than any other segment of the population, and it's difficult not to think that constantly keeping their lymph systems moving is one of the reasons why.[1] Their arm movements are extremely effective in mobilizing body fluids.

The effect of full moons on peoples' physiology is something I've experienced while being on call as a cardiologist. Can full moons actually alter one's physiology? I believe they can. As I personally saw, many heart arrythmias, hypertensive situations, and even a few heart attacks occurred during a full-moon cycle. Was it coincidence? Perhaps or perhaps not.

Is this theory scientifically proven? No, but if you consider that a full moon can move the tide 17 feet in the Bay of Fundy up in Canada, it stands to reason that it can also move the liquid in our bodies, which is made of mostly water. It's something I have thought about often.

The lunar rhythm takes its cue from the movements of the sun, Earth, and moon in relationship to each other, affecting everything from moods and menstruation to blood pressure and cardiovascular health. Together, they are constant reminders of life's pulsing rhythm that moves within and around us. When our rhythms are in sync, life flows easily. We have more energy and tend to view things more positively; we feel, think, and sleep better. When we're off balance, we succumb to ailments chronic and inflammatory in nature.

People who live off the grid today, who live as one with nature, experience the same sort of health benefits people around the world did millennia ago. Noted for their healthy diets, fondness for bathing in natural springs, and undeniable athletic prowess, the people of ancient Greece also followed environmental cycles while revering the deities they believed ruled the world. They looked to Gaia, the personification of the Earth, to help keep them healthy and hale, believing her to be a goddess who was the supreme nurturer and giver of life.

The ancient Greeks embraced the concept of a healthy mind in a healthy body, and their view of medicine incorporated both physical and mental well-being. The most famous and probably the most important medical figure in ancient Greece was

Hippocrates, renowned as the father of medicine for his insightful understanding of the human body. It is interesting to note that he was a big proponent of nature as healer, as the following quote attests: "Health is the expression of a harmonious balance between various components of man's nature, the environment and ways of life—nature is the physician of disease."[2]

So enamored with mind and body perfection, ancient Greece also gave rise to the Olympics, one of the biggest sporting events in the modern world. Godlike in stature and nature, the first Olympians showcased their indomitable athletic physiques in outdoor games played barefoot and in the buff, gaining strength and energy from their own training regimens and, in our opinion, their constant skin-to-soil contact with the Earth.

Their training included total-body workouts and various running exercises, including high-resistance running in sand to improve lower body fitness and aerobic performance—discharging toxins along the way. In addition to repetitive exercises, training also encompassed daily physical activities believed to enhance conditioning, such as digging, walking, hunting, and fishing, grounding activities we recommend today to keep your body balanced and in your health in top form.

When the athletes were not training, they rested, as this was part of a total regime that called for repose and sleep. They slept on animal hides or straw mattresses on the ground, materials that allow the transfer of Earth's energy into the body, and anointed themselves with plenty of olive oil to soothe the skin. Olive oil is a natural high-vibrational food that promotes good health while raising your body's energy, working in tandem with the energy of the Earth. Their diets were naturally organic, with whole grains and freshly picked fruits, nuts, and seeds, along with fresh fish and animal protein. Sunbathing was similarly recommended, not only to build endurance against the sun when they were performing in outdoor competitions, but also because solar rays were seen as beneficial to health. Energy from the sun is the original source of most of the energy found on Earth.

Soaking in the salt water, natural springs, and rivers was also part of their daily regimen, not only for cleaning but also for soothing tired muscles and inducing euphoria in the athlete: a kind of rejuvenating spa. Thermal baths in natural hot springs continue to be regarded today for their therapeutic properties, having been discovered and popular since the beginning of time. The bottom line, according to historians, was that the ancient Greek athletes were healthy and did not get sick easily. They stayed youthful into old age, which is evidence of the nutrients and grounding they enjoyed throughout their lives.

Headlining baseball news in the summer of 2021 showcased the daily health regime of one of the industry's ace pitchers, Adam Ottavino of the New York Mets, and it was remarkably similar to that of those first Olympians. Adam enjoys a healthy lifestyle that includes direct contact with the Earth's surface every day. His pre-game ritual includes walking atop the sacred ground of the nation's hallowed baseball stadiums, stretching in center field, and sitting on the dirt of the pitcher's mound for at least 15 minutes— shoes and socks off. In addition to tapping into the Earth's nourishing electrons, he believes he can connect with the energy the players of the past left behind.

"I feel like it's a sacred field," he told a newspaper reporter. "I want all the spirits that are in here to favor me. Whether it's real or not, I just try to act like it is."[3]

Follow the path of nomadic hunter-gatherers, ancient Greeks and Romans, and pilgrims on healing quests, and you'll discover sites designated as sacred ground all along the route of their journeys.

While walking here and there upon the Earth, these ancient people came upon mystic places that had a sense of heightened energy. The establishment of shrines during the Bronze and Dark Ages was very often at locations that had been venerated from earlier Neolithic times. The sanctuaries were placed at specific sites where the mysterious forces of the natural world were most accessible. This energy, stemming from the depths of the Earth, can be felt by the "psyche'" of man, raising feelings of joy, sadness, meditation, reflection, contact with the "divine" element, and ultimately, therapeutic energy of mental or physical healing. We refer to these as energy vortexes today, a swirling center of energy containing more Earthly energy than any normal place would.

Interestingly, these ancient sanctuaries were linked not only to specific places in the landscape but also to the movements of different celestial bodies such as the sun, moon, planets, and stars. They were situated at areas of landscape associated with the spirits and powers of nature. At first simple altars were set up to honor the spot, with buildings becoming more elaborate over time. What stayed the same, however, was the sacred space around these altars, which often included a cave, a running spring, a tree, or a stone—all of which, we know now, are great places to practice grounding.

Two thousand years ago, the Roman legions, wearied after battles, went out of their way to seek out sites renowned for their sacred energy to help heal their wounded comrades before making their way home. Churches were eventually built on these places, immersing their followers with the energy of the Earth during services. Step and Dr. Sinatra visited many of these churches when they were in Germany and France, taking the opportunity to connect to landscapes revered for their healing powers. "It was powerful to feel the energy of places that for centuries have soothed count-less souls," remembers Dr. Sinatra.

Step went even further when he walked on the hallowed paths of the Way of St. James in France in his quest to stay healthy after his near-fatal reaction to man-made electronic frequencies. What he experienced during his journey is what many seekers, past and present, hope for when taking a pilgrimage, which is the opportu-nity to connect with nature and the sacred energy of the Earth in places where it is most apparent. Historically the major motiva-tion of pilgrimages has been to seek healing. Pilgrims walked the Way of St. James, often for months and occasionally for years at a time, to arrive at the great church in the main square of Compostela in Spain and pay homage to St. James. Traditionally pilgrims lay their hands on the pillar just inside the doorway of the cathedral when they reach their destination. It is worn away in spots by the countless hands that have touched it over hundreds of years. Made of stone, the pillar is also a gateway to grounding.

As Step recalls, "Just like so many who walked this path, I could feel the spiritual connection with the living landscape I followed on my trek, relishing the slow pace of this journey. I feel that in Greece, too, where I live now. When I'm walking barefoot along the beach, grounding in the sand as I go, I reconnect to the natural rhythm that so many of us have lost in our modern-day, work-away world, where the tides and the season, not the clocks, become my reference point."

Step lived for a time in Baden-Baden, Germany, rediscover-ing the therapeutic effects of its natural hot springs. For centuries people looked to the sand and surf as a fully stocked pharmacy. As industrialization and city life took hold in 18th-century Europe, residents began to suffer from a mess of maladies, including diges-tive complaints and melancholia. Enlightenment physicians and researchers looked into the benefits of seaside living, which was positively associated with good health.

Their new wonder drug? Water.

A dip in cold seawater was often recommended for a number of ailments, as was a soak in thermally heated springs, which is among the most effective ways to immerse in the healing benefits of the Earth. Not surprisingly, grounding once again makes it appearance in medical annals of the past.

Traditional Chinese medicine holds that human beings replicate the universe in that both are made up of the constant interaction of five main elements: metal, fire, wood, water, and earth.[4] These five elements are believed to constantly interact with all of the organs of the body as the five phases of universal qi, or the life force—the intrinsic energy that travels along pathways in the body called meridians. Good health is achieved when the interactions between the elements are balanced and flow smoothly.

Eastern healing theory deems that disease occurs when the body is out of balance. Energy, if not flowing properly through the human body, will store negative patterns within it that can cause blockages. These blockages disrupt health, affect emotions, increase anxiety, deplete energy, invite pain, and trigger many other stressors that influence and lead to disease. Instead of treating the disease as is typical in traditional Western medicine today, Chinese medical practitioners, then and now, looked at the body as a whole rather than as individual symptoms. They strived to prevent disease before it began.

They did it—and still do—through ancient practices like Qigong and Tai Chi, both of which allow the body to balance itself for optimal health. Qigong typically involves moving meditation, coordinating slow, flowing movement, deep rhythmic breathing, and a calm meditative state of mind. It has been popularly referred to as Chinese yoga. Qigong is an integral part of traditional Chinese medicine, along with acupuncture, acupressure, and herbal medicine.

Tai Chi, a meditation in motion, was originally a form of martial arts. Today it is practiced as a form of whole-body movement that stimulates natural healing. By following age-old regimens like these, the body naturally rids itself of unwanted imbalances to efficiently function in harmony. Chinese medical practitioners also incorporate treatments like acupuncture to stimulate the flow of energy through the body by placing needles at specific points along pathways called meridians.[5] By stimulating these points, the body's qi, or vital energy, rebalances and restores the flow of energy.

Grounding activates and strengthens the Kidney energy—in traditional Chinese medicine this is thought to be the "root" or "core" energy for good health. Kidney energy correlates to and represents the life force. The more Kidney energy you have, the more stamina and resilience you'll have. When the Kidney energy is weak, it can lead to common physical health conditions such as painful backs or shoulders, arthritic or rheumatoid conditions, as well as more complex internal health problems. The first point of the Kidney Meridian, the entry point for qi, is located in the middle of the sole of your feet, a few inches below your toes, giving you direct access to the Earth's energy every time you walk on Earth, whether you are barefoot or wearing footwear that is conducive to the energy exchange of grounding.

Native Americans have always recognized the power of the land. We asked Lewis Mehl-Madrona, MD, PhD, of Cherokee and Lakota heritage, the author of several books (including the acclaimed Coyote trilogy, *Coyote Wisdom, The Power of Story in Healing; Coyote Healing, Miracles in Native Medicine;* and *Coyote*

Medicine, Lessons from Native American Healing) and a practicing physician with more than twenty years' experience in clinical, teaching, and research, what the Native American Indians knew about grounding.

He laughed, as did the tribal elders he posed the same question to, who, according to Mehl-Madrona, "laughed hysterically" at the notion of having to coin a phrase for this natural act. "We never had a term for it. No one talked about it. It's elemental. We just did it. I think you have to be non-grounded to think about grounding."

"Our ancestors in all Indigenous cultures knew that we belong to the Earth, as much as any rabbit or deer. Even our movements, our footsteps, honor the Earth. And the Earth honors us back. We are changed by a power that is not our own, an energy that transcends and understands us and engulfs us in its blessing. When we are in harmony with the Earth, our cells are in harmony with us. Harmony is the music of healing.

"Disharmony produced cellular degeneration, viral infection, and disease—AIDS, cancer, and so on. Never have we been so removed from the harmony of nature as today. One of our Navajo elders, a shaman and shepherd named Hosteen Begay, thought of asphalt as the curse of the *bellagana* (white man) because it prevents us from touching the Earth during the day. If we have lost our connection to the Earth, then we are not grounded, and we must endure, without protection, the lightning bolts flung our way. We are a part of the Earth and it is part of us."

Native Americans also naturally loved the soil. They sat or reclined on the ground with a feeling of being close to a mothering power. It was good for their skin to touch the earth. They wore leather hides and moccasins or walked with bare feet on the sacred earth. They built their teepees on the earth, and their altars were made of earth. This is why the old Native American still sits upon the earth instead of propping himself up and away from its life-giving forces.

In the southwest, Native Americans sought out spiritual vortexes, which today remain a draw for the health-minded visitor. Many are found in the energy field surrounding Sedona, Arizona, including Airport Mesa, Bell Rock, Cathedral Rock, and Boynton Canyon. The Navajo, Yavapai, and Hopi Indians long ago recognized the energy and spiritual power of Sedona's vortexes, honoring the land in this area and using the vortexes only for sacred ceremonies. According to visitors, some of the clues you notice when coming upon a vortex unexpectedly include feeling subtle energy vibrations such as tingling in the hands or buzzing throughout your body, and feeling hot or sensing a rush of energy or a shift in consciousness or perception. Often, the land will be very beautiful wherever there is a vortex, and trees may show twisting trunks and branches, spiraling in the energy field.

Other civilizations worshipped Mother Earth as well, giving her a range of different names. The Incans called her Pachamama, to the Aztecs she was Tonantzin. The Chinese Earth goddess is Hou Tu, and the Native American Pawnee tribes addressed her as Atira. In some cases, she predates writing. Prelinguistic references to her have been found, alongside shrines, statues, and paintings of her in every corner of the globe. She is the first goddess, the primeval one, the creator of all living beings.

Whatever name was bestowed upon her, it is evident that Earth has been recognized throughout time for her sacrosanct life-giving powers. You'll find references to Earth's sacred ground in the Bible in passages that instruct Moses and Joshua to "Remove your sandals from off your feet, for the place on which you are standing is holy ground" (Exodus 3 and Joshua 5:15).

Dr. Mehl-Madrona told us about a ninety-nine-year old Native American woman who lived alone on an isolated Indian reservation in Arizona. She lived in an abandoned railway boxcar without plumbing or electricity, with very few of the basic amenities we all take for granted. Her days consisted of tending her sheep, walking everywhere in her old leather moccasins, and thriving on food she grew. When she visited her doctor, she was lively, good-natured, and clear headed. She had sharp mental acuity and exuded overall well-being that belied her advanced age. How did she defy the odds and stay the picture of health despite her living conditions?

"She walked in beauty," Mehl-Madrona told us, explaining that it's a long-held belief of Native American culture that when you maintain a close connection to the Earth and live in harmony with the environment, you can achieve an ideal state of well-being and health.

Without artificial plastics, rubbers, and other synthetics used in footwear today, all of which has insulated us from the natural energy constantly emanating from the Earth, the ancients received a continuous gift of buzzing electrons that worked to revitalize every cell in their bodies. Whether they were searching for a better cave, hunting, gathering, planting, or simply sitting on the earth around the community fire, their bodies were constantly being replenished. This is part of our design, as natural as breathing, and it is available to all of us, anytime and everywhere. Synthetic soles on shoes today block us from Earth's healing energy.

So yes, shoes can make you sick. And from what we know now about grounding and health, this is just the beginning.

3

MAKING GROUNDING
THE ESSENCE OF MY LIFE

DR. SINATRA'S STORY

The two greatest environmental perils affecting our health today are being ungrounded and being bombarded by harmful frequencies in the electromagnetic fields (EMFs) in our 5G environment. Grounding mitigates both of them in ways that have changed my life forever.

I grew up in a diabetic family. My grandmother was diabetic. My mother became diabetic. And they both went blind. I was too young at the time to understand the reasons behind their illness, but I assume they contracted the disease from a combination of lifestyle choices, including diet and exercise—and genetics. As a child, I remember watching them succumb to the ravages of this condition as it slowly but surely robbed them of their vitality. They seemed to tire easily and often. They complained of headaches and constant hunger, no matter how much they ate. And their vision, blurry at best, gradually faded away until they could no longer see. That was a lot for a small child to take in, and I think their blindness frightened me the most. Would I go blind too? worried my thirteen-year-old self.

Turns out that was a valid concern. As a doctor, I know that mitochondrial DNA, and associated mitochondrial diseases, are transmitted through the mother. Mitochondrial genetics are really important when it comes to your health for it can give you a heads-up on any conditions that you could inherit from your mother. Diabetic vulnerability just happens to be one of the mitochondrial diseases that can be passed on from generation to generation.

Diabetes is also caused by lifestyle choices, with a steady diet of processed sugar and carbohydrates and inactivity both leading to weight gain. I tried hard to watch what I ate and how much I exercised, but more than that, I was constantly apprehensive about my eyes and I did everything and anything I could think of to ward off any potential blindness. I wore sunglasses all the time to protect my eyes against the sun's UV rays. I took supplements for healthy eyes, like Zeaxanthin, Astaxanthin, Omega-3s, and vitamins A and C, which can help maintain eye function, protect against harmful light, and reduce the development of age-related degenerative diseases of the eye. But deep down I was worried that no matter what I did, I was going to suffer from diabetic blindness at some point in my life due to a genetic predisposition.

Actually, my preoccupation with diabetes was one of the things that immediately gravitated me to grounding after learning about it from Clint Ober. I knew from my medical training and my practice that diabetes had been on the rise since 1950s. I hadn't yet discovered why until Clint told me his theory about grounding and illness and something inside of me clicked.

I hadn't heard of grounding, or "Earthing," as he called it, before I met him at a medical conference in 2001. He sought me out because of my background in cardiology and interest in electromedicine and asked if he could show me something. He had just completed his second study on grounding, which focused on studying how it affected cortisol and stress, and he wanted to discuss it with a medical professional.[1] What he said made a lot of sense to me right out of the gate and I wanted to learn more. I followed him to out to his mobile office where another medical doctor and a researcher were waiting. The researcher had developed a cuff that could measure blood vessel elasticity, and he and Cliff wanted to try it out on someone who would understand its importance. I held out my arm, interested to see if his device worked. Clint did the same. Blood vessel elasticity is an important part of cardiovascular health because you want your arteries to remain open and flexible to enable the blood to flow through them unimpeded. If they are rigid or constricted, it could lead to high blood pressure and arterial disease. My reading was good, but Clint's was better, and I wanted to know why. After all, I made it my life's mission to live and promote healthy living.

The reason, he explained, was grounding.

He shared his thoughts about walking barefoot on the earth and how it enables us to access healing energy from the Earth through an electron exchange that balanced the body. He spoke about how we are all energetic beings and how we are affected by electric energy, capturing my attention right away. Then he told me a story that stopped me in my tracks.

He spoke of the time he spent with Native Americans and how they used the Earth to help heal their illnesses, often digging trenches to bed the sick so they could heal in the arms of the Earth. He recalled hearing a friend's mother tell her son to take his shoes off. "Shoes will make you sick," she said. Then he explained how modern-day lifestyles—and synthetic shoes—have disconnected us from one of the most important healing sources on Earth—the Earth itself.

My initial impression of his hypothesis was that he was on to something incredible. Everything he said sounded very logical to me. And while I pressed him to spend time and money doing more research and conducting scientific studies so he and his theories would be taken seriously, I was with him from the get-go.

Through his discovery, I began to connect the dots about the rise of illnesses like diabetes that have affected so many of us in the last five decades. The numbers grew higher at about the same time we disconnected from the Earth by swapping our leather-soled dress shoes for the comfort and "style" of rubber-backed sneakers. I remember as a little kid walking to school wearing leather shoes and feeling great. People wore a lot of loafers back in those days, walking on sidewalks that were made out of conductive surfaces like natural stones and concrete, unknowingly keeping a lot of chronic illnesses at bay with every step. Interestingly, when shoe companies started manufacturing athletic footwear and expanded sneaker production in the 1950s, inflammatory illnesses like diabetes gained a foothold with its growth correlating to the growth of the sports shoe market (see the chart on the following page). Both of which were significant.

To my knowledge, we never had an exponential rise like this in diabetes before, and it was interesting to note that the more we became ungrounded and disconnected from the Earth, the more diabetes and other inflammatory illnesses increased. Today there are more than 130 million diabetics in this country.[2] That's one out of every 3.4 people. We know sugary food and a sedentary lifestyle contribute to this, but so does living ungrounded—the perfect storm for succumbing to this disease. It doesn't have to be this way, for many reasons. And grounding is one of them.

Several years ago, a team of Canadian researchers from Alberta Innovates-Technology Futures conducted an unpublished study they did on the topic of diabetes and grounding using rats as his subjects. Their goal was to show the correlation between being ungrounded, not exercising, and eating a diet of high-carb fast foods, a powerful combination that is contributing to the diabetic epidemic in the United States today, now more than 100 million strong. Rodents are particularly well suited for medical studies due to their anatomical, physiological, and genetic similarity to humans. In the study, all the rats in both the control group and the experimental group were given the same rat chow to eat, thus taking poor dietary habits out of the equation. One group of rats was kept in a cage fitted with grounding mats; the other group remained ungrounded. The researchers found that the grounded rats had consistently lower blood sugars than the ungrounded group in tests conducted over many months. Later, a human study done in Europe by the Polish researchers Karol Sokal, MD, PhD, and Pawel Sokal, MD, PhD, verified their findings.[3] With the incidences of diabetes rampant in the world today, the fact that grounding helps reduce and control blood sugar levels is huge.

As a doctor from a diabetic family, I found this result to be full of promise and vowed to make grounding an essential part of my life from that day on.

Grounding holds another fascination for me as well, especially in my career as a heart specialist. I've been studying energy medicine for decades. Pioneering works by Dr. Richard Gerber and W. Brugh Joy inspired me to learn more about these natural healing forces. As I found out through my own experiences and training in bioenergetics and metabolic cardiology, they were right on point. I treat my patients on a cellular level, focusing on energy-supplying nutrients that work throughout the body to charge up every cell so that it can function at optimal capacity. Grounding works with the electrical energy of the Earth to do just that for people, naturally.

Here's why. While many tend to think we are made up of flesh and bones, we are 60 percent water and are actually bioelectric beings in constant interaction with the environment around us. In fact, all living creatures are really a conglomeration of biological energy with low-level electrical currents running through their bodies to give them life. Our cells conduct electrical currents, resonating to certain frequencies in a continual exchange of energy. The elements in our bodies, like sodium, potassium, calcium, and magnesium, have a specific electrical charge. Almost all of our cells can use these charged elements, called ions, to generate electricity. People are constantly absorbing energy from the environment, including from light energy and their intake of oxygen, as well as from the food they consume. The body utilizes these outside sources of energy to create its own form of power, known as adenosine triphosphate (ATP), via the mitochondria of each cell. ATP is recognized as the energy of life or molecular currency, as it is responsible for powering the cells. The cells, in turn, generate the electrical current necessary for life, including recovering from injury and regeneration. We'll talk more about the science in a following chapter, but if you can picture your body with internal circuitry that's fueled by electrical cellular impulses, you'll better understand how it interacts with the Earth's energy.

The heart is an electrical organ powered by electrical signals from within the heart muscle that pump blood through the chambers of the heart and into your body. When these signals are interrupted, the heart may fail. In my work in cardiology, I see people "die" electrical deaths all the time. People go into ventricular fibrillation and have sudden cardiac death. Ventricular fibrillation (V-fib or VF) is an abnormal heart rhythm caused by disorganized electrical activity and leads to cardiac arrest. Without a heart rhythm, people perish quickly. When we shock them with a defibrillator and deliver a jolt of electric current to the heart, we can often bring them back. Conversely, if someone's heart starts racing in a panic, you shock the heart to make it stop beating. In that situation, shocking the heart restores its intrinsic electricity and it resumes a normal heartbeat. Believe me when I say that nobody understands the electrical nature of a human being more than a cardiologist. I am always curious to know more about energy and bioelectrical concepts that may be beneficial to the cardiovascular system.

While Clint Ober wasn't the first one to make the connection between the human body and the Earth's energy-giving surface, his research and clinical studies with regard to our health were the first to give it medical and scientific validity in today's environment. What he did was bring much-needed attention to the fact that there is an energetic phenomenon in our world that can either help or adversely affect our health.

The ancient Greeks were buzzing about the idea of energy and its direct impact on human beings, even giving a name to electricity, thousands of years ago. According to Merriam-Webster and other referenced sources, the term came from the classical Latin electrum, amber, from the Greek ἤλεκτρον (elektron), amber, which emitted static electricity when rubbed on other materials. The origin of the Greek word is unknown, but there is speculation that it might have come from the Phoenician word elekron, meaning "shining light."[4] As far as natural healing goes, the wisdom of the ancients still resonates today. In Western civilization, the first documented use of electricity to manage pain was by the physician Scribonius Largus in 46 AD. He claimed that just about every health ailment could be controlled by standing barefoot on a wet beach near an electric eel. Not surprisingly, finding dead electric eels on the beach is not an everyday occurrence, nor can it be something everyone can do every time they feel a headache or illness come on, but he was on to something that other scientists, including 20th-century researcher Robert Becker, MD, and Swedish professor Björn Nordenström, MD, elaborated on in extensive studies in the years that followed.

What they were all talking about then is what we call grounding today, a form of energy medicine that really works in our best interests. Disconnecting from this life-giving energy and living ungrounded, one of our greatest environmental perils, puts us at risk for an unhealthy future.

While the electrical activity from the Earth is beneficial, electromagnetic frequencies from man-made sources, including cellular technology and radio waves can be downright deadly. This is the second greatest environmental threat we face today.

One hundred years ago, an eminent Austrian researcher by the name of Rudolf Steiner wrote about the dangers that EMFs posed to humankind.[5] Like Richard Gerber, Steiner was a man way ahead of his time, writing about issues that affected humanity and spirituality long before anyone else considered them. Of these were his prescient concerns about unnatural waves of electricity and radio frequency. He urged caution toward this relatively new technology of the 1920s, telling people to beware of electricity and radio frequency, suggesting it may be harmful to our health. His fears turned out to be right on the mark. Now, one hundred years later, we are living in the 5G environment he warned about, where we are being bombarded by current levels of high radiation that are very detrimental to our physical, emotional, and mental health.

In my decades-long career as a cardiologist, I have put in at least five hundred emergency pacemakers in patients and performed thousands of cardiac angiograms. Of course, had I known about the potential dangers of X-rays and electrical frequencies, especially with my sensitivity to diabetic blindness, I would have always worn protective glasses before administering these procedures. But we didn't realize we needed to take extra precautions back then.

When I first started working with researchers to assess ongoing clinical studies on grounding and the environment, I learned first-hand just how invasive today's cellular technology could be on our health. Years after, we reported on blood viscosity after initiating a study on the outcome of grounding on blood viscosity at my office. Viscosity is an indication of the "thickness" of the blood, or its resistance to flowing normally. When the blood is thicker, it moves sluggishly, and there is an increased risk for red cells to adhere to one another and form clots. The heart has to work harder to pump the needed oxygen to the body. Blood viscosity can increase because of many factors, including medications, too many red blood cells, high lipid levels, conditions like diabetes and cancer, as well as certain environmental causes, as we were to find out.

Ten of us were participating in this informal study, most of us had medical backgrounds, and to begin, we all had our blood drawn. When we looked at our blood samples under a microscope, nine of us had thick blood with the consistency of ketchup, indicating a propensity for heart disease and diabetes. Only one of us had blood that looked like red wine. That person was Clint Ober, a man who had not only spent the last twenty years of his life grounding, but who also headed outside every 15 to 20 minutes in his bare feet to ground during our study.

When blood thickens like ketchup, it clots more easily and inflames the blood vessels, disrupting the blood flow so it can't do its work efficiently. It is the cardinal cardiovascular risk for heart disease. Blood with a normal consistency, more like red wine, allows it to move freely and quickly in the body, bringing oxygen to the tissues to keep the body in a healthy state.

What's interesting to note about this study is that we conducted it in a room with a hidden cordless telephone. None of
us knew that we were constantly exposed to its electromagnetic
frequencies. However, Clint was not exposed as much because
he kept walking outside to ground at least three or four times an
hour during the study. Our blood thickened, his remained fluid,
just like wine.

We were a health-conscious group so I couldn't help but
wonder if that cordless phone was putting out insidious, toxic
vibrations that were making our blood thick. When I started to
connect the dots, I asked everyone to go outside to get grounded.
We took our shoes off and walked on the grass and on the concrete, both conductive surfaces. We avoided walking on asphalt,
which blocks the flow of the Earth's electrons. Back inside, we
retested our blood, fascinated to discover that it went from red-
ketchup consistency to red wine. We followed this casual experience with a double-blind study with Gaétan Chevalier later on.[6]
We had twenty-four people in that study and the results showed
that after two hours of grounding, the blood thinned 270 percent.

The dangers of EMFs are unfortunately downplayed today,
in part, I believe, because people have become so dependent on
technology that they don't want to know of any potential problems with it. But it's time to acknowledge the truth. EMFs are
almost like a biological weapon in that we can't see, taste, or feel
them. Invisible, they are out there doing irreparable damage to
not only our health, but the health of future generations as well.
Cellular technology damages the mitochondrial DNA, the mitochondrial DNA that is passed from generation to generation, from
the grandmother to the mother to the daughter. There have been
studies about how harmful cell towers and power plants can be,
but for the most part, nobody is bringing it up.

I bring it up whenever I can and did so at a town council meeting in the Connecticut hamlet where I live. Town officials wanted to build a basketball court for residents, a worthy goal we all agreed. But it wasn't the basketball court that was the issue. It's where they wanted to put it that caused me to sound the alarm. There were about one hundred people in attendance, and I stood up and said that putting a basketball court next to an electrical power station was crazy. The officials countered that it was several yards away from the proposed building site.

Again, I told them it was not only a bad idea, but that it would put the health of our children and our community at risk. This was a very big electrical station, easily capable of emitting EMFs in abundance over a large area.

"Why would you want to do this?" I asked rather incredulously.

An engineer and another doctor he worked with who were in favor of the proposed location were quick to dismiss me, calling my fears unfounded quackery. The room started to buzz with muffled laughter, the kind you hear when people sense a nutcase in the room. Looking directly at the people in the audience, I responded, "Look, whatever you believe is your choice. But as a physician, I'll tell you this is not good."

The long and the short of it is that they put the basketball court there. Two years later, they suddenly took it down.

Cell phones, so much a part of our lives, also cause conditions that impact our health. When I first started practicing medicine, I would see fertility issues in the young women who came to my office. Men didn't seem to suffer infertility as much until, you guessed it, cell phone technology came into play.

If you're wondering why the switch, think about where men keep their cell phones. Usually, they carry them in the front pocket of their trousers. Now, you'll see infertile men all over the place and one of the reasons is 5G, 4G, 3G, and cellular phones. The data are alarming. After being exposed to cell phones for a few hours in such close proximity, sperm production goes down 400 percent. Ten years ago, Finnish researchers published a study about the sperm counts in 858 men, noting that they went down consistently in the 1970s and '80s.[7] Even then, the researchers concluded that this was environmental and surely preventable. Today male infertility is greater than the female, and sperm counts have declined by 50 percent over the last fifty years.

I am privy to studies like this because of my medical background, so I see what can happen when we are vulnerable to the toxins that are all around us. And EMF and living ungrounded are two of my biggest concerns.

You'll read more about the science and the stories in the following pages, from firsthand accounts of heart patients who turned their illnesses around by grounding to the heart-stopping story of my son's near fatal encounter with EMFs and his unwavering dedication to grounding.

But there is something we can all do now to take back our health. I have. And I've done it by making grounding the essence of my life.

As an aging man in my early seventies, I did what many people my age do; I moved to Florida to escape the winter weather of the north. I sold my house and built a condominium, steps from the beach. After I learned from the building engineers how I could build a special bathroom where I could be 100 percent grounded 100 percent of the time, I had one constructed in my new home. I walk excessively when I'm in Florida. I take advantage of long walks on the beach, I follow nature trails, I go fly fishing, you name it. As a result, I often get some tightness in my calves at night. These cramps can be very painful, and they are pretty disruptive to a good night's sleep. How do I deal with it? As soon as I get a cramp in my foot, usually in the middle of the night, I hobble to the bathroom and stand on my grounded bathroom floor. The discomfort goes away quickly.

Of course, you don't need to go to those lengths to live grounded. You can experience the beneficial effects of grounding wherever you live all year round. We'll tell you how in the following chapters. I live at the beach where I am fortunate to really benefit from the antioxidant effects of grounding every day. Add to that the fact that lightning strikes the ground in Florida on a near constant basis, charging it with billions of electrons. Here, whether you are walking outside on the beach, on the grass, atop surfaces made of concrete, ceramic tiles, or stones, you can absorb these electrons directly through your feet. And when you absorb them, it's like taking handfuls of antioxidants. It does the same job. Basically, you're attenuating the oxidative stress of the overactive autonomic nervous system.

Every morning that I can, I walk barefoot on the beach, burying my feet in the sand, then making my way to the shoreline, where the surf laps at my feet. Salt water is a great conductor of the Earth's energy, so walking in the water is one of the best ways to get grounded.

I also spend a lot of time in a small harborside town in Connecticut, population 6,600, where forested shores meet a freshwater river on three sides. Sidewalks wind past historic homes leading down to the harbor in one direction, or north, out of the village, onto wide, tree-lined avenues that spill into parks and conservation land. Walking here is a delight, and I make sure to get outside every chance I get, barefoot if I can, special grounding shoes on if I can't. I limit my exposure to technology and appliances, unplugging them when they are not in use, and make all my telephone calls on a landline. At night, I sleep grounded, too, with grounding sheets and bedding that enable me to connect to the Earth's surface from the comfort of my bedroom. Even when I travel, I bring grounding pads with me. I don't want to take a chance at sleeping ungrounded.

I have invested in a lot of grounding products over the years, finding them effective for those times when I can't get outdoors. Grounding products are made to connect to the Earth's energy when you plug them into grounded electrical outlets or use a ground rod system. Once they are connected, all you have to do is have direct skin contact with the products so that you can absorb the Earth's energy through them. Even when plugged into electrical outlets, they do not utilize any electricity. They simply conduct the Earth's natural energy through the ground wire of the grounded outlets. New products are being developed as we speak, making grounding without having to plug into an electric port very accessible.

I don't have cordless phones in my house. All my home computers are wired. You don't want wireless equipment near your body if you can avoid it, because the wirelessness itself can contribute to high blood pressure. People have difficulty sleeping because there are so many computers and cordless devices in their homes. No matter what technology exists in other parts of your house, we feel strongly that your bedroom has to be your castle. So in your bedroom, you don't want any stereos. You don't want cell phones or cordless phones or even a TV near where you sleep. You should sleep in a clean environment, free from technology if at all possible.

To enhance the effects of grounding, we also advocate staying away from processed foods, sugar, carbohydrates, and GMOs, and buying freshly grown organic produce whenever you can. I personally seek out high-vibrational fruits and vegetables, nutri-ent rich, and follow a Mediterranean diet. Doing so not only keeps my body healthy, it makes me feel great, too.

For many of us, grounding has become an antidote to pain, eliminating the need for toxic pharmaceutical drugs and reduc-ing our risk for these illnesses. Some commonly used pharma-ceuticals, although they have some beneficial effect, have been known to cause hypertension, especially in women, putting them at risk for heart disease, the leading cause of death in the United States today. Cancer, COVID-19, strokes, diabetes, chronic lung disease, and prescription drugs are also among the top causes of death in this country, and grounding can play a beneficial role in mitigating each of these.

I have looked at grounding from both a personal and a pro-fessional perspective for the last twenty years, weighing the risks and rewards involved in making it a part of a recommended health regimen. What I have discovered is that grounding helps rid us of accumulated negative energy and environmental toxins, boosts our immune system, and improves our overall health. I can say with all honesty that I believe grounding could be the most important heart-health breakthrough I've come across in my fifty years as a doctor.

We will explain why in more detail in the following chapters.

4

HOW GROUNDING WENT FROM LIFE CHANGING TO LIFE SAVING

SHARON WHITELEY'S STORY

If there's one thing I can say with certainty about my life's path, it's that it has always been about positivity, from my mindset to the products I've created and brought to market. I think that's why I was destined to meet Stephen Sinatra at a positive aging conference close to seventeen years ago, how I became immersed in grounding from the moment I stepped into it, and why I survived my heart attack, despite an ominous warning that I was 90 minutes away from certain death.

I've spent my life creating consumer products that promote positivity and well-being. I coined many motivational messages in an innovative company I founded, Peacock Papers, that were designed to inspire people to celebrate aging milestones with joy and strut their stuff by empowering them with original and upbeat sayings on greeting cards, party goods, and imprinted apparel for gift giving. It was the reverse of the "over the hill" negative phrases that were out in the market—still funny, but with a more positive spin. I conceived of and merchandised traditional pushcarts for pop-up vendors to display their wares with boutique-like panache just in time for them to be manufactured so they could contribute to the grand opening of Boston's legendary Faneuil Hall Marketplace. This mode of transitory merchandising became a staple in shopping centers worldwide thereafter.

Grounding shoes then became my passion with Pluggz close to fifteen years ago, followed more recently by Harmony783, both specialized shoe companies that pioneered a path into the wellness industry by helping people reconnect with the Earth's natural energy and get grounded through their feet in their everyday lives. Not only were these shoes "grounding," they were mechanically designed to be great shoes and very stylish ones at that! Let's face it, walking around barefoot is just not an option for many of us for several reasons. Safety from sharp objects lying in wait for an unsuspecting ground ambush is one; geography, hygiene, and foot comfort are others. Our inherent desire to look as fashionable and in style as possible is another factor, in spite of how our often-aching feet may feel in the process. I was motivated to help people reconnect, comfortably, with their former grounded selves—and walk their way into a healthier state. The flow of this revitalizing energy through your feet naturally gives your body what it needs to return to a more normalized body state.

I was almost simultaneously inspired to create TRU47, a company dedicated to innovating and manufacturing unique, pure silver–based antimicrobial germ-fighting products that manifested into a line of distinct and efficacious masks and protective face coverings, spritzes, sanitizers, and nasal inhalers during COVID days, and currently on my horizon, *functional fashion* apparel and wearable accessories to give consumers time-tested shields that protect their health safely against damaging EMFs and radiation impacts. As I fell further in love with silver, research ensued, and a custom-formulated line of pure organic essential oils imbued with colloidal and pure silver made its debut, extending immune-supporting benefits to pressed botanicals as they wafted through the air.

I never set out to create an enterprise, but I'd get tapped on the shoulder, stirred in the gut; my heart would go to my brain and it was more seductive than the sirens calling the sailors. I was also never drawn to anything "me, too, but different"—a repurposed iteration of an already created product. I was blessed with genes that magnetically attracted me to fresh, sustainably differentiated, and timely products people would value and love. It's in my DNA and I, along with my family, prove that entrepreneurs are to a great extent born, not made. Without sounding too woo-woo, it's my destiny. I am an identical twin, and my sister, Sheila Shechtman, and her two daughters have this same calling. Throughout my careers, I have responded to the zeitgeist of the times and brought to life innovative concepts, themes, and products that are right for that moment—or, truth be told, sometimes I've been a little too ahead of them—always original, and purposefully substantive. I am not interested in creating a nice want-to-have product with no value-based use. Nobody needs these today. Many successful entrepreneurs take an existing idea/product and build on that, but that's not been my life path. My mission is clear with my vision congealing and evolving further over time. Currently, that is a constant requirement; nothing remains static and entrepreneurial. Life is a living organism—it's organic. This drive is to help people take manageable and easy steps, grounded in science, to stay healthy—and do it as nature intended.

So how did I end up with a numbing chest pain that could have crushed all I have worked for? Stress likely was a factor at the time. Even though I believe in the upside of certain types of tension, this time it had probably gone too far. I had also been a smoker, an awful habit I picked up from my folks and by watching popular TV shows growing up where everybody, from the stars to extras ambling in the background, had a lit cigarette in hand. It was the epitome of cool—a statement that made you feel both *with it* and sophisticated. Unbeknownst to us back then, it was also deadly, and for me, a highly addictive drug. I empathize to this day with people who are afflicted.

I was one of those perennial, quit-then-start-up-again smokers, snuffing out my last cigarette with a vow to kick the habit for good, then yielding to the temptation again for any number of real or imagined excuses. I quit during college, and after my father passed away, picked it up all over again. I was in one of my this-is-my-last-cigarette phases just after I sold my shoe company, Pluggz, when I woke up in the middle of the night, sick to my stomach with the sensation that I had just gorged on a mile-long buffet and drunk a keg of beer (neither true, of course), dry heaving in vain. I got back into bed, slept on my grounding mat, and did some heart-centered breathing before I fell asleep. I woke in the morning feeling fine.

Two weeks later it happened again. This time, though, it was different. I felt a subtle residual pain in the heart area, more like a headache in my chest. It was not sharp or persistent the way I imagined a heart attack would present itself, so I really didn't give it much thought. My queasy stomach made me think I needed to toss my cookies, but like before, I was unsuccessful. There was nothing there to expel. I went back to bed where I meditated with some deep breathing and soon fell asleep on my grounding mat. I shooed away the thought that something was more awry in my body. I had people to see and places to go, and I couldn't be bothered with this nagging distraction.

In the morning, I woke up and headed off for a road trip to Colorado from my home in Arizona, stopping at my dealership for a quick car tune up before I set out for the long drive. The pain was still there, but my head was somewhere else. I tried ignoring it, surmising that it wasn't as if I was having a heart attack. As I pulled out from the car place, I noticed an Urgent Care sign glaring at me from across the street. I started to think about the long night ahead on dark roads and decided to stop in. Maybe it was just acid reflux, and I could get a quick prescription. I told the receptionist upon entry what was going on. They did an EKG and took some blood, ushering me into a patient room to wait for the results. They weren't long in coming.

"Your EKG is not conclusive," they informed me, "but your blood work is. As we speak, you are having a heart attack."

They sat me down and put an oxygen mask over my face. The next thing I knew they put me in the back of a fire truck ambulance. I called a friend of mine, Jean Reehl, who ran our fulfillment center and I said: "This is my twin sister's phone number. DO NOT call her now, just take her number down. I am on my way to the Tucson medical center." She said she would see me there and hung up.

When I arrived at the hospital, I was still standing, thanks to the oxygen they had given me. Waiting for me at the door with my friend Jean was a group of doctors, clipboards in hand. Among them was a cardiovascular surgeon who just happened to be on ER duty that night, which was very lucky for me.

"Normally," he said, "we would ask you about your life, your lifestyle, your diet, and do some more tests, including a stress test. But we think you have about 90 minutes left to live. Do you have a living will?"

I looked at Jean who was now in shock. "Make sure you have my sister's number but DO NOT call her," I said. I turned to the doctor and told him I didn't have a living will, adding emphatically, "Let it go on record here that I do not want to be a vegetable. Do nothing to resuscitate me, if I am otherwise 'gone.' Promise me."

I understood that this was serious and could go one of two ways—life or death—but I was relatively calm. It really didn't feel like a heart attack, at least not the kind I had expected from everything I had heard and read about them, and everything happened so fast. I told the doctors to go for it. Whatever happens will happen.

I woke up in the intensive care unit (ICU) and vaguely remember the doctors telling me that I now had a stent in one of my arteries and my echocardiogram showed that there didn't seem to be any permanent heart damage. I had beaten the odds. They kept me there for a day and half to check me, then kicked me out of ICU; a half a day later they sent me home and to rehab.

I had no history of bad cholesterol or high blood pressure. In fact, to the contrary, it was always low. Little did I know that my dad had cardiovascular disease. I wasn't aware of this important bit of family history. My parents were from a different era and back then, many didn't tell their kids their medical ailments. I do remember that when we used to go out together as a family on nature walks, I often saw my father pop a little white pill in his mouth—nitroglycerin, I later learned. I didn't know he had a heart problem. Yes, he was overweight, and in later years, he dropped the cigarettes but became a pipe smoker. He died at age sixty-two.

I went to rehab at Tucson Medical Center and then I went back to my life. I was a devoted proponent of grounding before my heart attack, thanks to Dr. Sinatra, and became an even bigger one after. I would go barefoot every single day that I could, and I would wear my grounding shoes—that I made—all the time.

I took bubble baths, leaving water to drip through the spigot—grounding me—and had pedicures, indulging in the pampering effects of grounding during these revitalizing soaks. I always slept grounded and woke up refreshed, and I continued to seek out more ways to maintain and improve my health.

As an older woman, I was determined to learn how to age not just gracefully, but gratefully and in good health. I signed up for the next Positive Aging Conference, the same conference where I had met Stephen Sinatra thirteen years before and first began my journey with grounding. I had already sold my footwear company Pluggz; however, I promised to help the new owners with their initial marketing efforts and happily set up and created a fun booth one last time. Steve Sinatra had a booth there as well with his new high-vibrational food company, Vervana. We talked about grounding, and I told him about my heart attack, adding that I believed what I learned about grounding from him all those years earlier saved my life. Serendipity at its finest. There are no accidents in my book. We became friends, colleagues, and now collaborators.

Steve told me that due to my blocked artery, now stented, I very well could have been having mini heart attacks all along, but my grounding practice probably kept me alive by keeping the blood flowing at least a little bit—enough. Grounding has been shown to improve blood viscosity, turning it from a ketchup thickness to a more fluid red wine consistency, which, in my case, I believe it did unequivocally. I will forever believe that I am here writing this book with the man who I consider saved my life.

Up until my heart attack, my ailments were seemingly minor. I had a benign cyst removed from one breast and remember the "teaching" Harvard doctor saying, "They are always bigger and deeper than you think," as he took out what looked like the raw end of a thumb. I suffered the loss of my voice permanently fifteen months post surgery. I then had an operation to artificially overcome a vocal chord paralysis resulting from a surgery that, as it turned out, was unnecessary. I went deaf in one ear at the same time until that was stented, and I was plagued with chronic circulation issues due to Raynaud's syndrome for as long as I could remember. No matter how intense or disabling they became, I conquered each of them without more surgery. My Raynaud's, a disorder which causes blood vessels to become narrow thereby limiting blood flow to affected areas like fingers and feet, is no match for the healing effects of grounding; I can restore circulation to my extremities by grounding each time. Now I breathe easier, knowing it was also the lifeline I needed to survive my heart attack.

At that conference where Dr. Sinatra and I reconnected, I had another chance meeting that led to the creation of a second grounding shoe company, Harmony783, when I was approached by a former Pluggz customer and investor who wanted to have more robust walking shoes, ones that were on my drawing board at Pluggz prior to my exiting the company. Our mission, from the start, was identical to Pluggz shoes—to help people reestablish the natural, healthful connection with the Earth that humans have enjoyed since day one simply by walking in shoes, which most of us do every single day. We chose the name Harmony to embrace the unadulterated, harmonious relationship between people and planet. The 783 part of the name relates to the energy frequency of the Earth at 7.83 Hz. Scientists call this the Schumann Resonance. Science shows that our brains, along with every other cell in our bodies, operate at a more optimal state when in contact with this harmonic resonance. We talk about the Schumann Resonance in more detail later in the book. It is a key part of every grounding story.

More reinforcing data about the benefits of grounding personally have since accrued. I dislocated my shoulder years ago on Vail Mountain and blew out my ACL on the hills of Aspen. I chose to do physical therapy instead of surgery and haven't had any trouble since. But now that I am living in a place where the walk up is like going up the Eiffel Tower, I decided to see an orthopedist to make sure nothing was amiss. I underwent a barrage of tests to rule out any developing ailments and to see if I was doing any damage to my knee and joints during my long walks home.

Upon reading my results, the doctor declared that I don't have a normal knee like others; however, he added he was surprised to find that I didn't have any arthritis either. Other medical tests also have shown that I have very little inflammation in my body—anywhere.

Can I also attribute my mobility and inflammation-free body to grounding? I absolutely believe I can. As Dr. Sinatra attests, it is the best antidote to inflammation that he has ever come across in fifty years of practicing medicine. I'm happy to be a poster child. I am also dedicated to creating as many new products as I can, enabling people to get grounded anywhere and everywhere without having to plug into a grounding port.

After building, from the ground up, six successful market-driven companies, earlier serving as the chair of the National Center on Women & Aging at Brandeis University, receiving numerous awards for business acumen, including Ernst & Young's regional *Entrepreneur of the Year Award* and other organizational and board affiliations, and after championing women in the pursuit of their entrepreneurial dreams, I am now more intent than ever on delivering beneficial products that speak to the needs of and empower today's more health-conscious and informed customers.

Aside from the inherent health benefits, I know from personal experience that grounding is beneficial for a reduction of inflammation, increased circulation, normalization of blood pressure, and a return to a more natural state of homeostasis (and possibly, it might save your life), while helping you feel more energized, balanced, and calm. It also helps banish the fatigue and the nagging aches and pains caused by inflammation that have become part of everyday life for so many of us over the years.

If grounding can help you reclaim that youthful barefoot bounce in your step as you step outside, wouldn't you want to do it every day?

5

ONE STEP FROM DEATH, A CANARY IN A COAL MINE

STEP SINATRA'S STORY

Three months out of college, I was trading stocks on Wall Street, embarking on a career I had dreamed of since I was twelve years old. I reveled in the music of the market, riding the highs with melodic precision, dancing through the downs like a ballerina on stage for her finest performance. I was born for this and I knew it. I worked on my own schedule, made my own rules, and did my own thing, relying on my intuitive lead to reach a level of personal success and satisfaction that, in this realm, was romance at its finest. In moments like these, my flow states were normal. I was in the zone, totally immersed and fully engaged in what I was doing. Laser focused and energized by the process, I was loving life and looking forward to all its possibilities. My health rocketed as my overall vibration was near the max. I rose and conquered day after day, feeling the rush of excitement and victory as I began depositing six-figure checks into the bank. I was thriving and living my passion and my dream.

That is, until I threw up on my keyboard with $15 million on the line. The market was in a panic sell mode, and it was only my fifth month at the helm.

Four years into my career, the stress of my trader's lifestyle began to take its toll. Instead of the active outdoor lifestyle I enjoyed in college, I spent each sedentary day surrounded by frenetic activity and computers, some nine or ten of them on my desk alone, screens flashing green and red and incessantly pulsing with a network of electric frequencies, not to mention the dozen or more that covered my co-workers' desks right next to me. There were fifty of us on the floor in those days, with wires running all over the place and underneath our feet, creating a magnetic field that was stealthily and silently working its way into my body and impacting my health.

I had no idea at that time.

My workdays, on average, were seventeen hours long, seven days a week, as I kept my finger on the pulse of current events and market fluctuations, even creating algorithms to profit on market moves. When I wasn't sitting in front of a computer, I was glued to my cellphones, often one on each ear. The stress was palpable. I seldom ate dinner before midnight, having little time or inclination to tend to my own needs during the day. Truth be told, I was not the normal trader. I was obsessed and intense.

I was aware what my lifestyle was doing to my health, but I planned to deal with it later. Not surprisingly, I started to lose weight, and my body began its slippery slide back down into the familiar state of illness that had plagued my childhood while dealing with mold illness. I went from superman on Wall Street to super sick in a matter of years. In time, my life became absolute torture. I receded from society. I looked sick. I was jaundiced, thin, feeble, and bone cold all the time. I stayed indoors, away from nature. Little did I know that as I was wheeling and dealing day and night, I was setting myself up for a deal breaker that left my life hanging by a thread until I was one breath away from death.

Unbeknownst to so many of us, disconnecting from the Earth's energy can take a toll on our health, causing a multitude of ailments that can be easily addressed by grounding. When you add in the unseen dangers of our modern-day environment, the effects can be deadly. I know because I became a case study for the hazards of toxic stress and tech overload. In fact, I was the veritable canary in the coal mine.

When I realized that I could no longer withstand the constant exposure to technology and stress, I quit my trading desk where I managed thirty young traders and moved to Boulder, Colorado—Boulder is an oasis of nature where the sun shines three hundred days a year with fresh mountain air and soul-stirring views nourish body and soul. My physical reaction to the stress of my Wall Street job and the electromagnetic frequencies that come with the territory was extreme. Most of my colleagues pursued their careers before burnout. But in the five years that I followed my dream, my body was wasting away—and I was only twenty-six years old!

After moving to Colorado, then Hawaii and California, to try to regain my health, I knew intuitively that I needed to get back to nature, to go mountain biking, to shift my life into another gear. What I didn't know was that all the technology I had installed in my new homes, top-tier Wi-Fi and cordless phones among them, was a big factor in my still-failing health. I had lost a considerable amount of weight on Wall Street during those last months on the job and was surprised to see it ticking down to 155, then 145 in Colorado, no matter what I did or ate. I just kept losing weight until I weighed in at 130 pounds sopping wet, and I was six feet tall.

Alarmed, I flew to Florida to check into a health clinic where I followed a strict raw diet. It was too little, too late. My weight plummeted as I dropped a staggering forty-five pounds in one month, about one third of my total body weight. I tried to visualize this in my head, picturing a stock chart with its gains and losses, upticks and downturns until it's something you no longer want to be a part of anymore. That's what my health looked like, a stock chart that was going down, seeing a precipice just before the bottom falls out. My health was on a downward trend for five or six years before it really hit bottom and sent me spiraling, like the stock market trending down before it crashes. That was my health chart.

The human body is amazing. It has evolved and adapted over millennia, enabling humans to survive and thrive despite devastating natural disasters and seismic ecological changes thanks to the healing resources found in nature. Modern-day lifestyles and super-charged technological advances have challenged the status quo, giving our health a run for the money.

I flew from Florida to a Texas clinic with my parents. It was critical that I receive an IV infusion immediately. The doctor who was treating me was a phenomenal doctor, but he was in over his head with this situation. He asked for my father's help as he struggled in vain to insert an IV line in my shrunken, paper-frail veins in an effort to get critically needed nourishment in my body. That's when my father jumped in. He arranged a private jet to fly us to a hospital in Connecticut that specialized in performing a risky cardiac procedure, one previously tested on newborn beagle puppies. It was being used as a life-saving treatment for premature babies in neonatal intensive care to get critically needed nourishment directly to the heart. It was rarely done on adults, but I fit all the parameters necessary to be one of the few—and time was running out. They had one bed left in the entire hospital when we arrived. I considered that to be a sign that I was in the right place at the right time.

I was in a state of shock when I was admitted, lying near death, up against impossible odds. I remember my mom and dad coming into the room where I lay virtually immobile in my bed. Literally two seconds before they arrived, a nurse was helping me try to urinate and all that came out was blood. I was covered in it. My mother could hardly move or speak and my dad looked shocked. I was surprisingly calm, thinking, "Wow, that's interesting." I instinctively knew at this point that I had to let go of the fear and find faith instead. I knew I had to surrender in that moment. I had been invincible on Wall Street, a fighter, and now I was vulnerable—and emotional. Emotions carry energetic frequencies that are key to healing. Consciously cultivating an emotion you want to experience can help transform your physical body and life experience.

The catheter came next in a traumatic procedure that scarred my bladder. The doctors who assessed the effects of that botched catherization were not optimistic about my ability to ever urinate on my own or have an erection for that matter. Here I was, just thirty years old, hearing words that emasculated me right there and then. I sat with their diagnosis for two seconds, before saying, "that's not an option." I didn't allow that pronouncement in my reality. I did regain normal function some three months later, fortunately disproving the doctors' grim prophecy about that and many other of my quickly failing capabilities.

But now I was frail, weak, and extremely dehydrated. I had pretty much lost all muscle function, so swallowing and breathing became extremely difficult. The doctors did not mince words. They took one look at me and said matter of factly that my chances for survival were slim and I had "a 1 percent chance of making it through the night."

I was acutely aware of what was happening. I could feel the pain, intense and relentless, but it felt like it was happening to someone else. It was surreal. In a near death experience, your life really does play out before your eyes. Years and emotions instantly flash by. You see everything that you've ever done in your life and you realize, in that moment, that you created everything that your life was. It was then that I had an epiphany. Here I was facing my worst fear, vulnerable and dying. It was like I was watching a movie where I was both the director and star actor. I somehow rationalized that if I could summon my biggest fear and manifest it, I could also realize my wildest dreams.

Physically, I was wasting away. The pain was intense. The doctors remained baffled by my symptoms and my rapid demise. I was teetering between life and death right before their eyes. They had never seen anything like this before. They just couldn't understand what was taking me down so fast.

They never found anything physically wrong. They couldn't attribute it to a disease or another condition. There was no illness, no leukemia, no cancer, no HIV, no Lyme disease, or the like. They ruled out every condition they could think of, checking me again and again with the same results.

I was in a free fall like stocks sometimes are, but it was my body, not my wallet, that was going bankrupt. To top it off, the energy of technology was so damaging to me during that time that it literally made me sick whenever I felt it near me; my body rejected it like kryptonite. Even 5 minutes on my laptop would fry my system and always triggered a setback in my recovery. I couldn't even look at a laptop; it literally made my stomach turn. I wanted to throw up just by having it in the bed with me. Any time anybody came into the room, I would tell them to turn their cell phones off.

I spent forty days in the hospital, fighting and battling to keep a pulse, trying to cleanse the toxins and technologies from my former life out of my new one, trying to regain a sense of wholeness and health again. My diet—spiritually, emotionally, mentally, and physically—focused on positive, high-vibrational nutrition full of life-giving energy.

My new understanding of the interactive force that surrounds us and flows through us, through everything, allowed me to rewrite the script of my experience and change the fiber of reality itself. Doctors told me I'd never be able to perform simple tasks on my own again, that I'd never be able to have a normal life, and I proved them wrong.

Recovery wasn't easy. Reclaiming my health, my independence, and finding a new normal was a full-time job and the focus of my life every day. Significant lifestyle changes were required to sustain any progress. The most significant ones? Disconnecting from technology and connecting to the Earth! I learned that you can't just stop the attack of bad energy, you have to replenish it with some other frequency. It's the synergy between the two that, in my case, made all the difference.

In spite of my intense spiritual experience during my illness, I still suffered from "tech withdrawal" upon returning to the outside world. When I was strong enough to start going out, I would watch others around me with cellphones on their ears and see how they appeared to be entranced, almost programmed. I remembered all too well when that was me. That kept me away from cell phones for a while—until that first iPhone came out. I was curious about all of the new features of this smart phone, and it reeled me back in. Resistance was futile. I became hooked and eventually my health began to suffer.

In the years since I had been in the hospital, I had regained my health. I was strong, and full of vim and vigor, almost like the old days, living my life's passion of travel and spiritual teachings. I was happy to be alive. I never returned to the city, opting for country life free from a daily assault of EMFs. Cities and the stress they exude were completely out of the picture for me then and still are. I knew there would be no more urban life in my future if I wanted to have any semblance of good health. Even living near the beach in Southern California became way too much for me. There were too many cars there, too many wireless technologies that got the better of me. I tried for years to deal with it but my sensitivities were too pervasive. After my near-death experience, all my senses became amplified. It was a blessing and a curse. Sounds and smells could be friendly if they were nature based, but man-made ones were agonizing to deal with. I craved nothing but nature. I couldn't get enough of it.

I finally moved to Napa Valley, in a canyon, and became a winemaker. I wanted to get my hands around something and create from a different level. I wanted out of technology and into the Earth. I found my calling when I found the grapes.

As my wine business grew, I started to resume my old habits, became glued to my iPhone, and chased success. I had a beautiful house, three cars, and was making good money. I was making a living off the land, with nature all around me. But then I started to get sick again. Smarter this time and not wanting to relive the horrors of my hospital days, I sold everything I could and gave away the rest. I began to make plans to go somewhere where I could reconnect with my spirit and the Earth full time. Impulsively, I booked a one-way ticket to France.

I followed a pilgrimage path that had guided seekers for centuries. I met fellow travelers as I walked, sharing tales and friendships on a weeklong journey that eventually inspired me to live in Europe. Once again, I didn't have a plan for where to go, but my intuition did, leading me directly to the healing waters of Baden-Baden in Germany's Black Forest.

My father told me about grounding as I was recuperating from my bout with death, explaining that one of the best places to access Earth's natural healing energy was in its lakes, seas, ponds, rivers, and springs. Baden-Baden's thermal springs enable you to ground all year round, even in winter, which was a big plus for moving there. I stayed for a couple of years, immersing in the beauty and bounty of this health-giving forested town, until it wasn't enough. I craved more interactions with nature and wanted to get in the most grounding I could every day.

Grounding is a potent antidote to the hazards of stress—and EMF exposure. Wireless mobile devices and Wi-Fi sources in our environment emit man-made electromagnetic fields, or EMF radiation for short. This unnatural form of EMF can cause a variety of stress-related responses in the body, like hypersensitivity, as it did in my case.

Studies indicate that when we constantly use mobile devices close to our bodies over long periods of time, exposure to EMF radiation can become harmful.[1] Studies have found links between EMF exposure and minor health concerns, such as headaches and skin rashes, to very serious concerns like the ones I faced. High concentrations of positive ions—also known as oxidants or free radicals—from EMFs can disrupt and interfere with our bodies' natural frequency on a cellular level. You simply can't thrive as well as possible when you're not communicating with the energy field of the Earth. When we are in direct contact with the surface of the Earth, like we are when we are grounding, negatively charged ions transfer into our bodies, which can help neutralize positively charged oxidants and keep our energy communication coherent and flowing. This can also help reduce inflammation and improve our overall feeling of wellness. While grounding cannot shield us from EMFs completely, we can take steps to minimize our exposure.

I currently live on an island in Greece where it's my goal to be as grounded as much as possible every single day. I focus on it as if I'm planning a nutritious meal and am always conscious of grounding anywhere I can get it, at any moment in time. I even connected a grounding rod made of copper and wire from the Mediterranean Sea all the way into my house so that I could sleep grounded at night. I no longer take chances with my health and I have grounding to thank for that.

I learned about the dangers of EMFs the hard way; now I experience an important first alert to a life-threatening danger. When I walk into a room I can feel if the energy is pleasant or nonharmonious. At my extreme sensitive state after the hospital, I began to become attuned to all sorts of electromagnetic information in the environment. I could sit down in a café and immediately sense the Wi-Fi network and could actually locate the router by closing my eyes and feeling the energy in my body. Most of the time this is not pleasant. I could sense strong cordless phones, booster devices, personal hotspots, and so much more. You know how you feel when you are in the presence of an angry charged individual who is negative. It's a feeling that you sense in your bones. This is just an example, but it shows that we can read energy and vibration with another sense if we attune to it.

You don't have to learn about the dangers of EMFs the way I did. Most people will never be as deathly sensitive to them as I am. But by disconnecting from technology whenever possible and connecting to the Earth as much as possible, you'll mitigate any possible effects on your own. We'll tell you more about the hazards of EMFs and the science behind them in a following chapter, along with ways to lessen their impact on your health. I'm still seeking out more ways to shelter from the perfect storm of harmful technologies I have faced in my life. More importantly, I have traded my own experiences for new role in teaching and empowering others to learn how to heal for free. And I've never felt better.

I made over a million dollars when I was twenty-four. It was the American dream fulfilled. But it took me down. During the next decade I spent all of that money and more searching for the answers for my health. At the end of the whole journey, I found that the best healing modality was right under my feet—and it was free.

6

THE SCIENCE, THE STUDIES, AND THE STORIES

Curiosity is an inherently human trait. It is in our DNA to question, explore, sample, test, and search for answers. We research, assess, and accumulate findings to develop reliable knowledge for just about every aspect of our lives so that we can be assured of increasingly accurate and trustworthy evidence to inform our decisions.

In business and in medicine, we rely on empirical data and proven explanations to guide us on our paths. Those of us in the health and wellness industry pay particular attention to multiple lines of evidence, drawn from observation, practices, and outcomes in clinical settings, as well as results from science-based studies, expert opinions, and feedback from a variety of targeted resources, including patients.

Research can provide important information about disease trends and risk factors, outcomes of treatment or public health interventions, functional abilities, patterns of care, and health care costs and use. The different approaches provide complementary insights. Clinical trials offer important information about the efficacy and adverse effects of medical interventions by controlling the variables that could impact the results of the study. And feedback from real-world clinical experience is crucial for comparing and improving the use of drugs, vaccines, medical devices, and diagnostics. By basing conclusions on evidence drawn from studies and observations, science can provide explanations that we can use to better inform our decision making.

We all shared our personal grounding stories in earlier chapters, documenting our belief in it with our own life's journeys, which support the evidence presented by some key clinical studies. Science backs up what we each experienced, but we believe that first-person testimonials also speak volumes about health initiatives that we consider effective.

Medical professionals like Dr. Sinatra rely on science to stay informed and educated about new types of treatments for any number of illness and conditions that may affect patient care. When he first started out, Dr. Sinatra followed conventional medical protocols when treating patients. It wasn't long before he became immersed in integrative medicine, thanks to a purely happenstance phone conversation initiated by one of his patients. He shared, "As I learned throughout my career, your patients are often your best teachers. They will come up with amazing discoveries that you may have never heard of."

Dr. Sinatra's first introduction to integrative medicine came about when a patient asked him to call a biochemist from Holland who had successfully treated his own arteriosclerosis with supplements, reversing plaque in his coronary arteries. He shared about Omega-3s, vitamin E, magnesium, phosphatidylserine, phosphatidylcholine, and other supplements that he knew little about at the time.

Ever since that conversation, Dr. Sinatra became a conventional-cardiologist-in-recovery, so to speak.

He turned my head and thus changed my life. I started to get involved with nutrition and food and vitamins and minerals. Then I went to a Gestalt psychotherapy training program. I studied with many psychotherapists from the West Coast and read a book by Alexander Lowen called *Bioenergetics*. That was one of my Eureka moments and I realized this might be the perfect fit for me as a heart specialist. Following on, I did a ten-year training program in bioenergetics and became a psychotherapist. When I was in training for psychotherapy, I realized that I was deficient in nutrition, so I took the board examination given by the American Board of Nutrition and I passed that. Around that time, I was working with the American Academy of Anti-Aging Medicine (A4M) and I completed my certification in anti-aging medicine. That's how my process evolved. I just starting taking more and more training in addition to contemporary cardiology. I branched out into other areas. I'm still going to conferences. It's amazing, I go to conferences to lecture, but lots of times I go to conferences just to learn.

That's actually how we all first heard about grounding and the studies that gave it validity, at conferences. We were not only intrigued by the findings and the stories we heard, but it all made sense to us too. We vowed to learn as much as we could about this "new" treatment, both professionally and personally, and have made it a part of our daily lives ever since.

The Science

Science isn't sexy, but sometimes you come across something that may change the game in radically shifting health on this planet and that can be incredibly exciting. Emerging science shows that direct contact with the ground allows you to receive an energy infusion, compliments of Mother Earth. Think of it anecdotally as "vitamin G" with the "G" standing for ground. Just as the sun above creates vitamin D in your body, the ground below provides you with a kind of electrical nutrition.

There is a constant rhythmic flow of this electrical energy in and around the Earth that is being continually replenished by the sun, lightning strikes, and heat from its always-hot molten core. In fair weather conditions, the surface of the Earth is negatively charged, letting a virtually limitless supply of free, unpaired electrons float through the ground. The atmosphere around the Earth is positively charged due to ionization by the sun's rays. In stormy weather, most lightning arises from a discharge of electrons from a thundercloud as they race back down to Earth.

The electron-rich natural rhythms of sunlight, lightning, and the Earth's hydrologic (water) cycle charge the Earth with an unlimited supply of negative ions. When we are disconnected from the Earth, our bioelectric potential is affected, leading to a cascade of debilitating health issues, with inflammation at the top of the list. When we reconnect with the Earth, our bodies begin an electron transfer that helps us reenergize and restore our body's natural balance. This energy infusion is so powerful! It can restore and stabilize the bioelectrical circuitry that governs your physiology and organs, harmonize your basic biological rhythms, boost self-healing mechanisms, reduce inflammation and pain, and improve your sleep and feeling of calmness. When these things happen, you feel better in a big way, even if it is subtle.

The Studies

Ongoing research provides intriguing evidence of significant physiological shifts in the direction of a revitalized and healthier functioning body generated simply by regularly walking barefoot or in special grounding shoes outdoors, swimming in natural bodies of water, gardening, and more or, while indoors, sleeping on a conductive bed mat, sitting/working with your feet on a conductive floor mat connected to the Earth via a wire, and many other ways. It's also as easy (and free) as taking a bath or standing in a shower while holding on to the metal faucet apparatuses at the same time.

Dr. Sinatra has collaborated in several pilot studies about grounding that have important implications. One in particular, on the electrodynamics (zeta potential) of blood cells, indicates that grounding can significantly improve viscosity (blood thickness), inflammation, and flow. There are clear indications that individuals with a variety of cardiovascular conditions may benefit greatly from staying in direct contact with the Earth.

This blood study entitled *Earthing (grounding) the human body reduces blood viscosity-a major factor in cardiovascular disease* by Gaetan Chevalier, Stephen T. Sinatra, James L. Oschman and Richard M. Delany, was published in February, 2013 and can be accessed online at PMID:22757749.

There are doctors and researchers in the medical arena that believe the blood viscosity study is Nobel Prize-worthy, especially in light of the health implications from COVID-19 when people were dying from blood clots. A new study[1] came out of Iraq during the pandemic found that people who were grounded survived the virus much better that those who weren't grounded, due to the fact that their lungs were not filling up with blood clots. This is meaningful research and further evidence of the benefits of being grounded.

Dr. Sinatra relays the following:

> When people get a coronary thrombosis, that means they have a clot in the blood vessels of their heart. If it happens in the brain, they call it a stroke. With COVID-19, multiple blood clots in the lungs could prove fatal in many instances. So basically, red ketchup blood is the zeitgeist of the times because red ketchup blood is the perfect storm for heart disease and health risks. What takes it away is grounding. It's

the natural antidote we lived with before the sneaker generation when rubber soled shoes disconnected us from Earth.

Now we have to get back to the grounded generation of earlier days so we can return our horrific red ketchup blood to red wine blood like it should be. How we do that is very simple, and the blood viscosity study proves it. This study shows that grounding had a very positive impact with a 283 percent reduction in blood viscosity.

Dr. Sinatra conducted thousands of angiograms on patients where he actually saw blood moving through their coronary arteries. He reported he would always be amazed at the patients whose arteries were 99.9 percent occluded. "It looked like a total blockage but there was a trifle of blood going through to keep person alive. That person was a ticking time bomb because any bit of added stress, including an emotional upset, bad news, or even cold weather stress, could cause a heart attack. This is where grounding is life saving and I just can't say enough about it. Whenever you put your feet on Mother Earth, you're recomposing your red ketchup blood into red wine blood and improving blood viscosity."

To reiterate, as Sharon can attest, grounding is a lifesaver for people with heart conditions. "I am convinced that I wouldn't be here today if I didn't practice grounding. It literally saved my life when I suffered my heart attack. I have a stent now that keeps my artery open and the blood flowing, which I have to believe has the consistency of red wine, not ketchup, thanks to grounding."

Bob Austin, a previous marketer for Healthy Directions, had a heart attack too and is here today to tell the story. He had read the grounding research conducted with Gaétan Chevalier, PhD, and other researchers and had often heard Dr. Sinatra talk about the benefits of grounding. Eight years ago he suffered a heart attack at four o'clock in the morning and immediately called 911. The first thing he did was chew on a baby aspirin before waiting outside for the ambulance, putting his bare feet right on the ground. Basically, he got "stented" right then and there, improving his blood viscosity himself by grounding. Like Sharon, he attributes grounding to saving his life during this emergency.

Another study Dr. Sinatra worked on showed how grounding can contribute to a destressing and balancing effect on the nervous system, and as a result, on heart function and heart rate variability (HRV). This study, published in *Integrative Medicine: A Clinician's Journal*, can also be read online at *imjournal.com*.

HRV plays a big role in evaluating the heart and determining your risk for future cardiac events. Your heart rate fluctuates with physical activity and your emotions; it is also affected by the time of day, the medications you take, the foods you eat, the food additives you may be exposed to, even electropollution. In this way, your heart rate is dynamic. It speeds up when you exert yourself or become stressed and slows back down with relaxation and sleep. That's normal.

HRV represents an accurate assessment of your ability to cope with both internal and external environmental changes. Decreased HRV—having too "fixed" a heart rate interval—is now regarded as the most accurate reflector of personal stress and even a predictor of sudden cardiac death. In fact, altered HRV has been accepted as a risk factor for sudden cardiac death that is independent of all the other usual American Heart Association heart risk factors, such as age, chronic hypertension, diabetes, smoking, and so on.

Medications can decrease HRV as can overexposure to the electropollution of radiofrequency from cell towers, cordless telephones, and cell phones, something we'll address in a following chapter. Electromagnetic disturbances can also push those people vulnerable to low HRV to develop cardiac arrhythmia, stroke, and sudden cardiac death. Electro-sensitive people report cardiac arrhythmias as one of many symptoms they experience with exposure to hazardous unseen frequencies.

People with low HRV are often less able to "go with the flow" when faced with external stressors and more prone to stress-related disorders such as cardiovascular problems. The good news is that if you can increase your HRV, you can reduce the likelihood of stress-related disorders, including cardiovascular disease and sudden cardiac death. Our study on HRV showed that grounding can help improve it, as can Tai Chi, yoga, Pilates, relaxation, and simple physical activity like taking a walk.

There were twenty-seven individuals in the study who each had marked improvements in HRV after just twenty minutes of grounding and who continued to improve the more time they spent grounded. In patients who experience anxiety, emotional stress, panic, fear, and/or symptoms of autonomic dystonia, including headaches, cardiac palpitations, and dizziness, grounding could be a very realistic therapy. These patients may see positive effects, most likely within twenty to thirty minutes, and in almost all cases, in forty minutes.

In addition to the two important studies noted that have indicated improved cardiovascular and rheological (blood viscosity) dynamics, including autonomic nervous system regulation, another study[2] that should be mentioned is one conducted by Gaétan Chevalier, PhD. This study was undertaken to determine if grounding can also rejuvenate your skin and facial appearance. The immediate results speak volumes.

In this study, forty participants were observed for sixty minutes. Some were grounded; others were not. A Laser Speckle

Contrast Imaging (LSCI) camera continuously and non-invasively recorded changes in their facial blood flow. The results were surprising. Just one hour of grounding restored facial blood flow regulation and enhanced the repair of skin tissue in the participants, leading to improved facial appearance and other implications of overall health, like relief from aches and pains.

Remember, Sharon Whiteley suffered from Raynaud's Syndrome, a seasonal circulatory affliction that restricts blood flow, especially in the fingers, toes, and face.

> Raynaud's causes blood vessels to constrict in response to cold, stress, or emotional upset. My fingers and toes turn white as they numb out, then get all pins and needle prickly and uncomfortable. While not life threatening, this condition is definitely a pain to live with, pun intended! Some people I know who are afflicted with it have a hard time handling refrigerated items as their fingers chill out and lose feeling at the most inopportune times. How I handle it is what anyone with this condition should do; get outside and sit on the ground, touching the Earth with your bare hands or feet if the weather permits. After a short time outside, your white finger tips will come to life with color, as will your cheeks, and the numbness will subside. If you can't get outside, simply hold onto the neck of a faucet and let the water, preferably warm, run for up to fifteen minutes. That's also an easy way to tap into the healing effects of grounding inside your home or office!

Inspired by her cold feet—and most of all, the indisputable scientific basis behind the benefits of grounding she first learned about during a lecture by Dr. Sinatra, then studied and came to champion—Sharon started a shoe company called Pluggz, manufacturing grounding shoes that were conductive to the Earth's energy due to a custom formulated carbon plug that was embedded in the soles. Before she stepped out with her shoes, she commissioned a study to test the efficacy of the revolutionary plug technology and its ability to permit the shoe's wearer to get grounded as they walked.

In her placebo-controlled, IRB (International Research Board) protocoled, single-blind pilot study, subjects were assessed after baseline measures were taken on the physiological changes that were produced by wearing Pluggz shoes for a period of only ten minutes.[3] Using Gas Discharge Visualization (GDV) devices, Thought Technology ProCom, Physiology Suite with BioGraph Infinity, and CardioPro software, significant changes in heart, head, thyroid, adrenal, and lumbar responses were detected. Taken as a whole, these changes are indicative of the body's relaxation response.

"The data shows the early markers of the onset of a relaxation response," said Melinda Conner, PhD, who is the chief investigator at Optimal Healing Research, the independent researching firm retained to oversee the study. "In addition, the increase in spectral brightness in the fingers and hands indicate improved electro-dermal skin response"[4]—probably due to an increase in circulation.

Conner added that findings from this pilot were particularly significant because the subjects were tested for only ten minutes in a dry desert ground that has relatively poor continuity with the conductive part of the Earth's surface. There was not an ounce of moisture in the ground, a contributing factor to becoming grounded. Sharon went on to continue the evolution of conductive footwear in another company, Harmony783.

Disconnecting from the Earth also causes sleep and mood disturbances as demonstrated in a study on cortisol by Gaétan Chevalier.[5] When you ground, you regulate your cortisol dynamics. In other words, you get more of a circadian curve with cortisol. Remember cortisol is the hormone of vigilance, like you are waiting for the other shoe to drop. Grounding regulates hormones. Your hormones respond to your autonomic nervous system, communicating back and forth and helping regulate homeostasis in the body. In other words, grounding is the best way to get the body in sync with the nervous system.

In this study, twelve participants with complaints of sleep dysfunction, pain, and stress were grounded to Earth during sleep in their own beds using a special conductive mattress pad for eight weeks. Eleven of twelve participants reported falling asleep more quickly, and all twelve reported waking up fewer times at night. Grounding the body at night during sleep also appeared to positively affect morning fatigue levels, daytime energy, and nighttime pain levels.

We all sleep grounded now as a matter of course, even taking our grounding pads with us on the road. Sleep plays a vital role in good health and well-being throughout your life, helping protect your mental and physical health and overall quality of life.

Another meaningful and less-popularized study that had significant implications in the health of people of all ages was one conducted at Penn State College of Medicine on grounding and preterm infants.[6] Research in adults has indicated that electromagnetic exposure affects the vagus nerve. However, how it plays out for the most vulnerable babies is also noteworthy. The vagus nerve is the longest nerve of the autonomic nervous system (ANS) and is one of the most important nerves in the body as it helps to regulate the body's physiology. ANS activity is outside of our conscious control. The ANS is responsible for managing our breathing, heart rate, body temperature, digestion, and other basic processes necessary for survival. The vagus nerve system also acts to counterbalance the fight or flight system and can trigger a relaxation response in our body.

"Preterm babies in the NICU have a lot of health challenges due to the immaturity of their lungs, of their bowel and of all their organs, so we decided to look at how electrical grounding could help improve vagal tone and mitigate some of those challenges," said Dr. Charles Palmer, professor of pediatrics and chief of new-born medicine at Penn State Children's Hospital, who helped manage the study. "Anything we might do to improve the babies' resilience would be good."[7]

What they concluded by the study was that a baby's ANS is able to sense the electrical environment and the baby seems to be more relaxed when grounded. According to Penn State College of Medicine researchers, "electrical grounding" improves their health outcomes.[8]

Stress reduction and relaxation are key to optimal heath for all of us and one of the best ways to do both is by grounding. Gaetan Chevalier, K. Mori, and James Oschman published a study in the journal *European Biology and Bioelectromagnetics*, that concluded that the simple act of grounding reduces overall stress and tension.[9] There were fifty-eight subjects in the study, the majority of whom showed marked positive changes in EEG, EMG, and pulse rates after grounding. In fact, half the subjects showed rapid improvement in these readings as soon as they were grounded.

Not surprisingly, one of the biggest health elephants in the living room of the world right now is high blood pressure. The COVID pandemic is also one of the reasons so many people are suffering from anxiety, depression, and stress, factors that increase blood pressure.

Dr. Sinatra assisted Dr. Howard Elkin with a study on how grounding affects blood pressure.[10] There were twelve participants in the study, all of whom were on one to three hypertensive drugs.

They were able to reduce their blood pressure medications or even get them off of them altogether by grounding for up to twelve hours a day. It is interesting to note that all twelve participants, 100 percent of them, had some degree of blood pressure lowering with grounding. This is significant because high blood pressure is so prevalent in our society today, especially on the heels of COVID-19.

Intuitively, Dr. Sinatra felt that grounding would lower blood pressure because it does everything right for the body. Now we have proof. "Grounding lowers what we refer to as the sympathetic drive. The sympathetic nervous system (SNS) is the part of the automatic nervous system (ANS) that revs things up. The parasympathetic nervous system calms things down. When the ANS is in balance, all is well. But when the SNS goes into overdrive, like when we are worried, angry, sad, distressed, illness can happen. I've always believed that emotionality affects our health and it just makes sense that lowering SNS activation leads to optimum health."

Speaking of stresses such as the kind the pandemic assaulted us with, the study we mentioned earlier that was conducted in Iraq pointed to grounding as a healing mechanism in the treatment of fifty-nine COVID-19 patients. In that study, they put grounding patches on the chests of a group of people who were ill with COVID-19 and compared them with a group of ill people who were not grounded. The ones who were grounded fared much better than the patients who were not grounded because their lungs were much freer from blood clots. This study, by Dr. Haiswe Abdul-Lateef Mousa, MB, ChB, MSc, included results that showed that after one to three days of grounding, most patients experienced improvement of the following symptoms: fever, dyspnea, cough, weakness, headache, chest pain, taste and smell loss, anorexia, and body pain. The researcher concluded that grounding showed significant curing and preventative effects in the treatment of COVID-19.[11]

We all need to take a conscious timeout and get back to nature. The simple practice of grounding contributes significantly to discharging much of that negative energy and toxic material. People who are not privy to the benefits of grounding may chalk up their anxiety, anger, and feelings of depression to stress, not understanding what else may be causing them to feel uneasy and have all the negative energy.

We know, from the science, the studies, and the stories, that when you are disconnected from Earth, your well-being, physically, mentally, and spiritually, is impacted.

The Stories

Stories about the healing effects of grounding abound, taking on new momentum as more and more people become aware of it and begin to incorporate it in their daily regimens. Our own stories are poignant testimony to the fact that grounding made us feel better—and in some cases saved our lives. There are many more we've encountered in our quest to spread the word about.

Suzanne Somers, celebrity and author of more than twenty-six books on health and wellness, is also an advocate for clean, non-toxic living. She has made it a mission to take on those invisible toxins that are changing the way we live and feel and offer us alternatives that will let us reclaim our bodies and health again. She is passionate about educating and informing the public about the dangers of chemicals and environmental hazards that plague people of all ages and has aligned with the top integrative medical professionals to discover what we can do about them. Over the years, Dr. Sinatra has become one of her go-to experts, teachers, and good luck charms for his insights and advice on keeping the body healthy.

"I learned about grounding from Dr. Stephen Sinatra who has collaborated with me on a number of my books. It's funny how we don't realize the extent to which we are disconnected from the Earth and our shoes are even part of the problem. I never thought about what that meant in terms of our health. It's actually similar to a lot of other technological advances we initially think are great but that actually contribute to the weakening of the human body. I remember when we used to make a sticky paste of Ivory soap and water to get rid of ants in our kitchen. Then one day my father came home with a new way to get rid of ants fast, a deadly can of Raid. We sprayed the whole baseboard of our kitchen, inside the cabinets and out. Then he started spraying outside of the house so the ants would not come it. I believe that chemical fixes as such were the beginning of a lot of our health problems. It seems so obvious now. But when you look at something as benign as rubber-soled tennis shoes, who knew what that would do to the human body in terms of health. Very few people wear pure leather-soled moccasins, naturally conductive, anymore. Unfortunately, the major athletic craze and all the variations thereof that boasted high-performance rubber soles—all non-conductive—fundamentally changed the electrical system of the body. The connection from the electrical of the Earth to the electrical of the body was disrupted and it has affected people's energy in ways we don't even yet realize. I don't think this subject has been explored so deeply to know that this is the root of other diseases we haven't even thought about."

"When Dr. Sinatra first explained grounding to me," she continued, Suzanne decided to try it. "I began to incorporate grounding in my own life and have really noticed the difference, especially in the quality of my sleep. In addition to getting grounded as much as possible during the day, I always sleep grounded now. But last year I experienced terrible injuries from a bad fall and grounding was not only a big part of my recovery, it was life-saving.

"My husband and I were on our way out one evening and I was waiting for him at the top of our stone stairs, some twenty or so steps. He grabbed my hand as he always does and his foot slipped on a boulder. He went down and I went down on top of him, except that my head banged into the ground beneath me full force and the torque of that made me hit my forehead on another rock. I didn't realize that in that fall I had broken my neck and spine and fractured my hip and my jaw. I was in bed for a full year. Part of my recovery was sleeping grounded. I had heard from Dr. Elkin and Dr. Sinatra that sleeping grounded would speed up my recovery. I was told at that time that I was not far away from becoming a total paraplegic. Now I'm being told that I am nothing short of a miracle.

"I think grounding was a big part of it. I think it restored the electricity to my body and along with my dedication to physical therapy, it helped me overcome the odds. I'm back to around 97 percent today. And it's even hard to remember the last year. It was always in my brain that I was going to be well."

Stories about athletes grounding abound in the news, from football legend Aaron Rodgers' preference for sleeping grounded to Red Sox pitcher Adam Ottavino's pre-game ritual of walking the ballfield barefoot before he throws the first pitch. Elite Tour de France cyclists have touted the accelerated recovery and healing effects of grounding for their injuries, regularly turning to its inflammation-fighting properties to relieve swelling and torn muscles.

Nature loving celebrities have gotten into the act, claiming their devotion to Mother Nature and natural good-for-you lifestyle choices. Naomie Harris, one of the stars of *Skyfall*, turns to grounding to counteract the effects of jet lag from cross-country and international flights that transcend time zones, as do Michael Gelb, author of *How to Think Like Leonardo da Vinci* and *The Art of Connection*, and Bulletproof founder, Dave Asprey. Others regularly exercise outdoors, benefitting from grounding through such practices as Tai Chi, yoga, Qigong, and more.

A family member was stricken with debilitating pain in his abdomen one Thanksgiving. At the time, he was admitted to Middlesex Hospital in Connecticut with an acute abdomen. He had gone through previous surgery on his gut, about twenty years earlier. Whenever you have surgery on the abdomen, you can develop adhesions that impact your bowel and cause painful, often life-threatening obstructions. The doctors at the hospital told him he needed surgery to relieve his agonizing pain.

"I went to see him in the hospital," Dr. Sinatra recalled. "The surgeons were putting off the surgery because it was Thanksgiving weekend. He had tubes attached to his body and he was bloated and miserable. I noticed that he was on an electric orthopedic bed, which had a steel triangle hooked up to a steel chain that was hooked up to the steel bed. I remember saying to myself, I wonder if this bed is grounded, because of all the metal. I strongly suggested that he hold on to the steel triangle as much as possible while he was awake. In my previous research, we demonstrated significant blood thinning, and I surmised that if better circulation and blood flow could be achieved in GI tissues, perhaps that could facilitate enough energy to get the bowel adhesions to open up.

"And guess what? His whole GI tract opened up! He started to pass gas, then he started to burp, releasing everything that had been previously blocked. He ended up not having the surgery after all. His surgeon was indeed perplexed. He had a mile-wide smile on his face because he was so grateful to get through this horrible weekend without being cut open. His doctors couldn't believe that this guy cured himself. I will never forget it and neither will the doctors who treated him! To me, it was another grounding miracle."

7

HUMAN SUSTAINABILITY

THE FOUR Rs OF BETTER HEALTH

What does sustainability mean to you? For us, sustainability is about people and their well-being and providing solutions that help all generations, present and future, live a healthy and happy life. As wellness specialists, we have a theory about living your best life. It's all about restoring your health, recharging your energy, and revitalizing your body the way nature intended. As grounding enthusiasts, we believe it begins with one easy step—reconnecting with the Earth.

In the two+ million years that modern humans have inhabited the Earth, we have gone from a nomadic hunter-gatherer society that survived primarily by hunting, trapping, fishing, and gathering edible plants to pastoral groups that raised animals for transportation and food to horticultural and agrarian communities that cultivated the crops we grew to sustain us. The common denominator was the land we relied on in order to thrive. Even when we established our first cities and towns, we settled where the land was fertile and water was nearby. In those days, people remained in direct contact with the life-giving Earth. They had their hands in the soil as they worked the fields, planted crops, and picked tree-ripened fruit. They were physically active. They walked everywhere, sometimes barefoot, sometimes wearing footwear made of animal hides. They fished and washed in rivers, streams, and lakes. They slept under the stars or in shelters devoid of electricity. They breathed in clean air and they ate nature-made organic food free of modern-day miracle formulations and chemically induced additives. They fortified their bodies with nourishing herbs and plants rich with vitamins, antioxidants, and protective polyphenols and phytosterols that can lower cholesterol levels and reduce inflammation. The diseases that felled them were infectious in nature and not like the non-communicable diseases (NCD) we face today.

What's different now?

Throughout history, people have been drawn to cities as centers of trade, culture, education, and economic opportunity. Up until the 1800s, the vast majority of people still lived in mostly rural areas. But by 1900, after the onset of the Industrial Revolution, when people began working at factories and moving into the cities en masse, they created urban areas that paved over the lands they once couldn't live without. Urban population growth was fueled by new technologies, most notably ones that enabled cities to build upward. Innovations in steel enabled the development of skyscrapers, which allowed for greater population densities. And, of course, the invention of the elevator made it possible for skyscrapers to take people upward, higher and higher and away from the Earth, to their soaring suites and offices in the sky.

Experts say that over half of the world's population today lives in densely populated urban areas and that around two-thirds of people will be living in cities by 2050. Megacities, where wireless automation is king, are fast becoming the next big thing as people crowd into ever-larger urban centers with a population of ten million or more.

But what's the cost of this new technologically oriented life, and is it sustainable for our health going forward? Unfortunately for all the advances humankind now enjoys, we've seemingly gone backward in terms of our health. And much of this decline points back to our lost connection with the naturally nourishing electrons found on the surface of the Earth.

Humans are now living longer than ever, with average life expectancy across the globe shooting up from about fifty years old or so during the 20th century to about seventy-two years in 2022, according to the World Health Organization (WHO). The WHO now predicts global life expectancy for women in places like the United States to soar to eight-five years in another thirty years. The boost in life expectancy could be linked to significant advances in medicine, better sanitation, and access to clean water. Although all of these factors have also greatly reduced mortality rates from infectious diseases, the deaths from chronic degenerative diseases such as Alzheimer's, heart disease, and cancer have been on the rise. In other words, people are living longer and are dying from different diseases than they did in the past.

"An American baby born in the year 2000 can expect to live seventy-seven years and will most likely die from cardiovascular disease or cancer," writes anthropologist Dr. Barry Bogin.[1] An expert in human physical growth and development, nutritional ecology, evolutionary biology, Maya people, and human adaptation, he is the author of more than 230 books, articles, book chapters, and popular essays on the topic, including *Patterns of Human Growth*, 3rd edition (2021), *Human Variability and Plasticity*,

Human Biology: An Evolutionary and Biocultural Approach, and *The Growth of Humanity*.

As is often the case with biological advantages that humans sometimes gain, old age also comes with trade-offs, which, in the case of our current disconnection from Earth, is not surprising.

The remarkable improvements in life expectancy over the past century were part of a shift in the leading causes of disease and death. At the dawn of the 20th century, the major health threats were infectious and parasitic diseases that most often claimed the lives of infants and children. Currently, noncommunicable diseases that more commonly affect adults and older people impose the greatest burden on global health.

Which begs the question. How do we sustain our health for the long term?

The answer, to some degree, depends on lifestyle choices that are able to restore our health, recharge our energy, and revitalize our bodies.

Start by restoring your health

Restoring your health means reducing the causes behind the chronic conditions we suffer from today. Take heart disease, for example. Along with cancer, cardiovascular disease is arguably the number one killer of people today. What causes heart disease? There are a number of factors involved, but stress, diet, and exercise play important roles here.

While there are several forms of heart disease, the most common form is coronary artery disease (CAD), which is a narrowing or blockage of the blood vessels in the heart—also called atherosclerosis. When the arteries that bring blood to your heart muscle harden and narrow, coronary artery disease occurs. Left untreated, CAD can lead to arrhythmias, heart failure, and a heart attack. When it comes to heart disease, many people—doctors included—focus on cholesterol. But the truth is, cholesterol is not the only thing that contributes to heart disease. Nor is sugar singularly responsible for diabetes. As in the case of heart disease, research suggests that inflammation inside the body plays a role in the development of type 2 diabetes.[2] Stress is another significant contributor to many of the ailments we see today, as is high blood pressure and inactivity. Each of these is relatively new in terms of the medical issues that have plagued us through time. And as we have discussed, each can be traced to our disconnected lifestyles from Earth's surface and, to some degree, our constant connection to wireless technology.

Dozens of studies on grounding have proven beyond a doubt that grounding has significant positive effects on our physiology and heart health. Grounding's many physical benefits—particularly those that lead to a healthy heart—include a decrease in inflammation and an improvement or elimination of the symptoms associated with many inflammation-related disorders; lowered stress and increased calmness in the body by moderating heart rate variability, nervous system activity, and stress hormone secretion; improved efficiency of the cardiovascular, respiratory, circulatory, and nervous systems; a reduction in chronic pain—and better sleep.

To begin the process of restoring our health, we need to address the health conditions that are all too prevalent in today's modern society. They include the following:

Inflammation. It's one of the top risk factors for heart disease, and a much more accurate predictor of a future cardiac event than high cholesterol levels. As you've read in previous chapters, inflammation is the culprit behind most of the chronic diseases we face today and is a key by-product of our disconnected lifestyles. Grounding helps mitigate it.

Inactivity. Not getting enough physical activity can lead to heart disease—even for people who have no other risk factors. It can also increase the likelihood of developing other heart disease risk factors, including obesity, high blood pressure, high blood cholesterol, and type 2 diabetes. In looking at how to prevent heart disease, walking is an excellent option. Walking for just thirty minutes four times a week can go a long way toward minimizing your risk factors for heart disease, and when you walk grounded, the benefits increase significantly.

Uncontrolled High Blood Pressure. When your blood pressure is elevated, it can cause the inner layer of your arteries (called the endothelium) to become damaged. When this happens, your body sends cholesterol to plug up the damage. Over time, this cholesterol forms plaque that narrows and hardens your arteries—setting the stage for heart disease. However, high blood pressure is a risk factor for more than heart disease. It can quietly damage the body for years before symptoms develop. Uncontrolled high blood pressure can lead to disability, a poor quality of life, or even heart failure or a stroke. It can damage and narrow your arteries, limiting the blood flow throughout the body. Over time, as it weakens the arteries, it can form a bulge (aneurism) that may rupture and cause internal bleeding. It also affects the brain because it too depends on a nourishing blood supply to work properly. Hardened arteries or blood clots caused by high blood pressure can cause strokes and varying degrees of cognitive impairment. Kidneys also require healthy blood vessels to help filter excess fluid and waste from the blood. High blood pressure can damage the blood vessels in and leading to the kidneys. Having diabetes in addition to high blood pressure can worsen the damage. Many people do not realize that the combination can damage the eyes and contribute to sexual dysfunction, too, all because of damaged arteries and limited blood flow. What helps to alleviate this all-too-common condition? Regular exercise, weight loss, stress relief, a healthy diet—and grounding.

One of the most powerful benefits of grounding is how it helps reduce blood pressure. As many of you know, high blood pressure may be related to "hyperviscosity," which means your blood is thick and sticky and moves slowly through your circulatory system. In other words, your blood is thick like ketchup, and that feeds the inflammation process that damages arteries, boosts blood pressure, and increases the risk of blood clots.

Chronic Stress. When looking at the risk factors for heart disease, many people (doctors included), overlook stress. But stress is a significant contributor. When you're stressed, your body reacts by releasing stress biochemicals like adrenaline—increasing your heart rate and raising your blood pressure. If this occurs on a regular basis, it can lead to high blood pressure and heart disease. Stress can also worsen or increase the risk of conditions like obesity, Alzheimer's disease, diabetes, depression, gastrointestinal problems, and asthma. When stress does occur, it's important to engage in stress reducing activities—such as yoga, meditation, and, you guessed it, grounding.

We've all heard people tell us not to stress about the things that worry us and keep us awake at night. Sure, that's great advice, but putting it into practice is the challenging part. When people tell someone not to stress about something, they usually refer to stress's emotional or psychological effects. Common synonyms of the phrase might be "chill out" or simply "relax." What they're saying is, "don't worry." But that is not the way we are designed. We do worry. Worry (or stress) plays a vital part in our body's internal warning system producing the fight-or-flight response. However, there is a marked difference between the stress reflex that comes from fleeing danger and the emotional stressors of daily life. One could help save your life; the other could end it.

Since stress can be so subjective, stress triggers can vary from person to person. Even so, some stressors are generally common to all. Stress can be acute, like with the fight-or-flight response, or chronic. Chronic stress comes from the demands of daily life. This type could prove dangerous to our health if left uncontrolled. While it's unrealistic to suggest that you can eliminate stress from your life completely, you can try techniques to improve your body's response to stress. For instance, try five minutes of deep breathing every morning, listen to relaxing music on your way to work, meditate in nature, or take a walk with a friend or your pet, making sure you are grounding while you do so. We've found that grounding not only makes the day feel less stressful as we regain our footing and find our balance, our energy level is noticeably higher. Grounding can work the same magic for you.

Keep your body's energy recharged

Now that you have turned to grounding to help restore your health, use it to recharge your body, too. From keeping your energy levels at their best during the day to getting a valuable good night's rest, grounding works wonders.

Exercise. If you have a chronic condition, regular exercise can help you manage symptoms and improve your health. Even twenty minutes of exercise a day can do wonders for your body and mind as it helps release feel-good endorphins. Walking, dancing, swimming—anything physical that you enjoy—are good ways to exercise. Exercise increases blood flow throughout the body, helps modulate metabolism, improves mood, and even supercharges mitochondria, which are your cellular engines. All of these benefits can help to counter low energy levels. What we've found to be very important for exercise success is committing to a specific exercise schedule. Blocking out time will help you stick to your exercise commitment.

Aerobic exercise can help improve your heart health and endurance and aid in weight loss.

Strength training can improve muscle strength and endurance, make it easier to do daily activities, slow disease-related declines in muscle strength, and provide stability to joints.

Flexibility exercises may help your joints have optimal range of motion so they can function best, and stability exercises may help reduce the risk of falls.

Adopting a simple weight-training program can also benefit those with cardiovascular health concerns. Studies indicate that strength training can also lower blood pressure, decrease cholesterol, and increase cardiovascular endurance.

Plus, if you can exercise outdoors while grounding—simply by keeping your feet, barefoot or while wearing conductive footwear, planted on the ground—it can be doubly refreshing. You'll be recharging your body with the Earth's energy field while also taking advantage of the inherent health benefits of grounding such as reducing inflammation and blood viscosity, increasing blood flow, and reducing any pain you may be having.

How Exercise Helps Your Health

- **Heart disease.** Recent studies have shown that mild exercise training is often tolerated well in people with heart disease, and it can produce significant benefits. For people with high blood pressure, exercise can lower your risk of dying of heart disease and lower the risk of heart disease progressing.

- **Diabetes.** Regular exercise can help insulin more effectively lower your blood sugar level. Physical activity can also help you control your weight and boost your energy. If you have type 2 diabetes, exercise can lower your risk of dying of heart disease.

- **Asthma.** Exercise can help control the frequency and severity of asthma attacks.

- **Back pain.** Regular low-impact aerobic activities can increase strength and endurance in your back and improve muscle function. Abdominal and back muscle exercises (core-strengthening exercises) may help reduce symptoms by strengthening the muscles around your spine.

- **Arthritis.** Exercise can reduce pain, help maintain muscle strength in affected joints, and reduce joint stiffness. It can also improve physical function and quality of life for people who have arthritis.

- **Cancer.** Exercise can improve the quality of life for people who've had cancer, and it can also improve their fitness. Exercise can also lower the risk of dying from breast, colorectal, and prostate cancer.

- **Dementia.** Exercise can improve cognition in people with dementia, and people who are active on a regular basis are at less risk of dementia and cognitive impairment.

Sleep is the time when our bodies do the hard work of detoxifying, restoring, and rejuvenating. Researchers once thought that lack of sleep primarily affected cognitive health—with symptoms of tiredness, inattentiveness, and poor cognition. But more recent studies have revealed that chronic sleep deprivation can also increase your risk of obesity, diabetes, cardiovascular disease, and even early death!

When it comes to maintaining a healthy body, most people know they should eat healthy, exercise, and avoid smoking. But what few people know is that sleep directly impacts your health and your heart. A lack of sleep can lead to a heart attack or stroke and can increase your risk of developing atherosclerosis and high blood pressure. A new study, published in the *European Heart Journal, Digital Health* November 2021, found that going to bed between ten to eleven o'clock PM is linked with a lower risk of developing heart disease compared to earlier or later bedtimes.[3] The researchers found that the rate of heart disease was highest in people who went to bed at midnight or later. You need at least seven hours of sleep a night. But according to the Centers for Disease Control and Prevention (CDC), more than one in three American adults say they don't get this much. The American Heart Association also says that people who sleep less than six hours a night are at a higher risk for high blood pressure.

The impact of sleep length on heart health has been proven in numerous clinical studies. In a study published in the *European Heart Journal*, researchers examined the sleep habits of 475,000 participants in fifteen previous studies.[4] What they found is that chronic sleep deprivation—less than six hours a night—raised the risk of developing or dying from heart disease by 48 percent and stroke by 15 percent! It showed that fifty-year-old men who get five hours (or less) of sleep each night were twice as likely to have a significant cardiovascular event within the next two decades than those who got seven to eight hours of sleep each night.

A lack of sleep is also strongly associated with diabetes, which can contribute to heart disease. In a study published in the *Annals of*

Epidemiology, researchers at the State University of New York and the Warwick Medical School determined that people who slept less than six hours a night were more likely to have impaired fasting glucose—which can lead to diabetes—than those who slept six to eight hours a night.[5]

When you're sleep deprived, your body produces less of the satiety chemical leptin, the messenger that tells you you're full. So, if you're not sleeping enough, you're more likely to eat more, which can contribute to weight gain, diabetes, and heart disease. A chronic lack of sleep also heightens your sympathetic tone, raising your levels of stress hormones that contribute to heart attack, stroke, and high blood pressure. Plus, while you sleep, your blood pressure is naturally lower, so not sleeping enough can keep your blood pressure elevated for more time throughout the day.

Sleep needs can vary from person to person, but in general you want to strive to consistently get between seven to eight hours of sleep each night. Avoid screen time, including phone, laptop, and television, before turning in. Keep your bedroom cool and dark. This environment is best for proper production of melatonin— your primary sleep hormone—as well as for keeping your nasal passages moist for optimal nighttime breathing. Remember to remove all offending EMFs from your bedroom as they interfere with sleep and can lower your sleep-producing melatonin. And make sure to practice grounding during the day so your body is relaxed and stress free for a good night's rest.

By definition, sleeping is an unconscious activity, so you may wonder how it's even possible to stop the tensing of your muscles at night. Grounding has a calming effect on the entire body. Specifically, it's been proven to slow down the sympathetic nervous system and reduce cortisol levels, two major factors that drive muscle tension. Chronic elevation of cortisol disrupts our circadian rhythms and affects our ability to sleep. It has also been linked to inflammatory pain and depression, and it increases our risk of chronic conditions such as hypertension and arrhythmias, and even sudden death. By encouraging parasympathetic branch activity, grounding helps people relax and reduce stress. Grounding has a balancing effect on your body's automatic nervous system (ANS)—a control system for the body. The ANS functions without you having to think about it and controls your internal organs. It affects your heart rate, digestion, respiration rate, and more; it also leads to normalization of cortisol levels and improved heart rate variability.

In a study by researchers Maurice Ghalay and Dale Teplitz of twelve individuals with sleep disorders, pain, and stress, sleeping on a grounding mattress pad for eight weeks restored the subjects' day-night cortisol secretion to normal.[6] The majority also reported better sleep as well as less fatigue, pain, and emotional stress.

Ongoing research by Harvard Medical School cites that a sleep shortfall interferes with the normal function of the brain's house cleaning system.[7] In the deepest sleep phases, cerebrospinal fluid rushes through the brain, sweeping away beta-amyloid protein linked to brain cell damage. Without a good night's sleep, this housecleaning process is less thorough, allowing the protein to accumulate—and inflammation to develop. Then, a vicious cycle sets in. Beta-amyloid buildup in the brain's frontal lobe starts to impair deeper, non-REM slow-wave sleep. This damage makes it harder both to sleep and to retain and consolidate memories.

Just one night of lost sleep can keep beta-amyloid levels higher than usual. The problem is not so much a single night's poor sleep, which you can compensate for, but a cumulative pattern of sleep loss, leading to decreases in the structural integrity, size, and function of brain regions like the thalamus and hippocampus, which are especially vulnerable to damage during the early stages of Alzheimer's disease.

Take steps to revitalize your body every day

Grounding and interacting with nature every day is the best way to revitalize your body. Get outside as often as you can, hiking on dirt trails, swimming in ponds, rivers, lakes, or the salty sea, reading a book as you lean against a tree. Plant a garden and get your hands dirty. Take a nap on a sandy beach or a grassy knoll. Head to the park for a jog in special grounding shoes. Go off the beaten path and find a rock where you sit and contemplate nature. Bring your yoga practice outside. Join a Tai Chi class on a grassy lawn. Meditate as you sit on the ground. Walk in the woods with your dog, petting your pooch to get grounded as you go. Breathe fresh air. Disconnect from technology and reconnect with the surface of the Earth and revitalize body and soul. It's the easiest way to revitalize yourself wherever in the world you are. And best of all, you'll heal for free.

In addition to grounding every day, it is important to fortify your body. Eat an anti-inflammatory diet like the Pan Asian Modified Mediterranean Diet (PAMM), which combines the best foods from the traditional Japanese and Mediterranean cultures, both known for their health and longevity. With the PAMM diet, you can eat moderate amounts of saturated fats from eggs, avocado, and animal protein. Plus, you want to limit (or better yet eliminate) sugar, white flours, and other simple carbohydrates that can lead to inflammation. Instead fill your diet with vegetables, legumes, fresh fruits, lean proteins, cold-water fish such as wild-caught salmon, and olive oil, the secret sauce of a healthful diet. People who live in the Mediterranean basin, like in Portugal, Spain, and Italy, and who consume extra virgin olive oil on a daily basis lead the world in longevity. The science is simple. Olive oil is rich in polyphenols that support healthy cholesterol dynamics and reduce proinflammatory gene expression. Eating the PAMM way is anti-inflammatory because it limits your body's insulin response, minimizes harmful free radicals, and gives you lots of fiber to quickly move toxins and food through your digestive tract.

Stay hydrated. Your body depends on water to survive. Every cell, tissue, and organ in your body needs water to work properly. For example, your body uses water to maintain its temperature, remove waste, and lubricate your joints. Water is needed for overall good health and you should drink a good amount of water every day. Most people have been told they should drink six to eight eight-ounce glasses of water each day. While plain water is best for staying hydrated, other drinks and foods can help, too. Fruit and vegetable juices, milk, and herbal teas add to the amount of water you get each day.

Interestingly, water may be used to ground in the same way the physical Earth is used for grounding. Simply wading in a clear lake or swimming in the ocean is a good way to ground yourself. As always, be sure to stay safe when swimming, especially in murky or deep waters. The ocean is full of dissolved salts and minerals and represents a superb conductive medium for grounding. Similarly, lakes and rivers, while generally containing fewer minerals and salts than the ocean, are still good conductors. If you are near mineral hot springs, take the opportunity to soak in the high mineral and salt content found in them; these are great places to get grounded.

If you have a salt water pool and the water is in contact with a metal drain pipe going into the ground, you'll be able to ground while swimming. Normal tap water in a pool can also be conductive, but again, it needs to be in contact with a metal fixture going into the ground. If you don't live near water or it's too cold to enjoy a swim in a pool, take a bath or a shower, or even hold onto a metal faucet while the water is running. Tap water contains minerals and salts and is conductive, but it must be running through metal pipes that go into the ground in order to ground you.

Detox. Hands down, environmental toxicity is one of the biggest health challenges we face today. Herbicides, BPA, and other chemicals that nature never intended are permeating our food and water supply, our lawns, our personal care products, and our homes. Not to mention the EMFs we discussed earlier. But don't let this bring you down.

Toxins are natural and foreign substances found in the environment and are normal byproducts of cell metabolism. Our bodies are designed to process and eliminate toxins through healthy organ function and detoxification mechanisms. However, since the Industrial Revolution and the introduction of chemical fertilizers and pesticides, the level of toxins present in our air, water, and soil has skyrocketed to unprecedented levels. Heavy metals such as mercury, pesticides such as DDT, and xenoestrogens such as phthalates found in plastics have infiltrated our environments and, ultimately, our bodies. This massive increase in environmental toxins has put tremendous strain on our cells' detoxification mechanisms, and consequently, we store the toxins rather than excrete them. Wireless radiation and electromagnetic fields generated from electrical devices are other sources of toxins. These invisible toxins are quite harmful and impossible to completely eliminate, so reducing exposure is important.

In addition to grounding, you can prevent toxins from building up and disrupting physiology through lifestyle modification, exercise, healthy organic foods, and herbal supplements.

The simplest way to start is to do what comes naturally. Breathe. Your lungs are considered one of the largest detox organs. With every inhalation, oxygen enters our lungs, and with every exhalation carbon dioxide is expelled. Our bodies, on a cellular level, are doing the exact same thing—bringing in nutrients like oxygen and expelling wastes like carbon dioxide.

Taking a few moments out of your day to consciously breathe, especially while sitting on the Earth and grounding, can alleviate stress and help in the detoxification process. Find a quiet space, sit with a straight spine, and breathe in and breathe out slowly through your nostrils. Feel the air entering and exiting your nose, and when thoughts begin to enter, remember to focus on the breath again. Regularly practicing conscious breathing will likely improve all aspects of your health.

With detox, take a double-down approach. Do your best to avoid toxins, and help your body get rid of the ones you are exposed to. Your hard-working body eliminates toxins in four ways: through your GI tract, lungs, urine, and sweat. The less toxic your body is, the easier it is for your detox organs to do their jobs.

One of the best ways to detox is to simply reduce the amount of chemicals you eat and absorb. Choose whole foods, organic is best, whenever you can. Buy cosmetic products that contain fewer chemicals and more natural, organic ingredients. Stay away from pesticides, and don't use harsh chemical cleaners around your house.

If it's processed, avoid it—processed foods use chemical preservatives. Eat natural, whole foods like fresh fruits and vegetables, eggs, unprocessed nuts, seeds, and yogurt. If it's mass-farmed or GMO, avoid it—the odds are high that herbicides and pesticides were liberally used while it was growing. Stick to small, local farms as much as possible. Buy from farmer's markets, where you can ask growers how they treat their crops; you'll have a much better shot of dodging chemicals.

Avoid added sugars, which can cause inflammation through-out your tissues and organs. Inflamed cells are stressed cells—they won't work nearly as well as healthy cells. Grounding when sup-ported by a nutritional diet does wonders for your health.

Approach your detox as more of a way of life, starting with your daily diet and your exposure to EMFs. Eat lots and lots of fiber-rich foods, especially organic vegetables and fruits. A fiber-rich diet not only speeds up digestion and helps you flush tox-ins from your body, it can help you lose, or maintain, a healthy weight, too—a win-win for health.

Another one of the best ways to detox is through regular exer-cise. Exercising every day will help increase circulation and nutri-ent flow and decrease the toxic load. If you are not keen on going to the gym to exercise, schedule at least a thirty-minute grounding walk each and every day. Another way to increase circulation is through use of a sauna or, better yet, soak in thermal springs if you can. As mentioned previously, the skin is one of our primary organs of elimination, so using a sauna regularly is a wonderful way to sweat out toxins we accumulate on a daily basis. Start off with a low temperature and duration of exposure, and work your way up to increase sweating. Remember to drink plenty of water with electrolytes before and after the sauna to mobilize toxins and pre-vent dehydration.

Sit in the sun for a few minutes. Vital for maintaining healthy bones, vitamin D is crucial for calcium absorption, which is why low levels can lead to increased risk of osteoporosis and weak bones. The most natural and efficient way for your body to make vitamin D is via sunshine-on-skin, though taking supplements can help, too. Prevention packs a powerful punch. Start early to best keep bone loss at bay. The best way to impact your bone health is by getting enough vitamin D. Another smart move? Weight-bearing exercises like walking, jogging, or jumping rope are also bone strengthening and something you can do while grounding!

Take small steps. Choose achievable goals and set realistic expectations. Be mindful of what's good for you and the planet. We are always mindful of the carbon footprint we leave behind and take steps to reduce, recycle, and reuse materials when possible. Just as we avoid artificial barriers when we are grounding, including plastics, rubbers, and other synthetics that insulate us from the natural energy emanating from the Earth, we try to avoid or limit our use of materials that contain Bisphenol A (BPA)—a chemical used to harden plastic. It is found in countless consumer products, including plastic cups, plates, bottles, storage containers, toys, and packaging, to name a few. You simply can't avoid it completely, but there are steps you can take to protect yourself from the most common causes of BPA exposure.

- **Avoid plastics whenever possible.** Just get rid of as much of it as you can—cups, plates, utensils, storage containers, etc. Use glass, stainless steel, ceramic, or porcelain containers to store food. Avoid drinking water bottled in disposable or reusable plastic. Plastics are as terrible for the environment as drinking from them is for you. Reusable glass or unlined food-grade stainless steel water bottles are readily available online and at big-box stores.

- **Don't heat plastics.** This has been shown to degrade the plastic, allowing even more BPA to leech into food. Reheat food the old-fashioned way—on a baking sheet in the oven. You shouldn't use microwave ovens; in fact, throw them out with your cordless phones because they both can emit harmful radiation. If you do have any plastics, hand wash them instead of putting them in the dishwasher.

- **Avoid or limit canned food.** Fresh fruits and veggies should always be your top choice, and frozen is the next best option. For other prepackaged foods, search for those that are sold in glass jars or cardboard brick-shaped cartons. Also, avoid sodas and other canned beverages. They have absolutely no nutritional benefit, and most soda cans have a BPA lining to prevent the beverage from taking on a metallic taste.

Keeping your environment as healthy as possible will not only help sustain the Earth, it will also help sustain the health of all living things that depend on the health benefits the Earth provides through grounding.

8

DO NO HARM

One of the oldest binding documents in history and considered to be the gold standard in medical ethics for some 2,500 years is the Hippocratic Oath, which is still held sacred by physicians who pledge their commitment to the highest medical ethical conduct during their career.[1]

Dr. Sinatra remembers taking a modified version of the oath when he graduated from medical school more than fifty years ago, "solemnly promising to do no harm, to treat my patients to the best of my ability, to respect patient confidentiality and to teach the secrets of medicine to the next generation. All of which I strive to do as a doctor, keynote speaker and author."

But lately, medicine is shifting. The practice of medicine is becoming more fast paced and less personal, with doctors often seeing patients in time-limited slots. Additionally, we have adopted a medical approach that has led to a worrisome expectation that there is a "pill for every ill."

We have seen a dramatic increase in chronic ailments and diseases over the last few decades, making both patients and their doctors anxious to speed up the healing process and improve their health and happiness. How are they doing this? By prescribing medications and the quick fixes their patients are looking for.

Too often this leads to prescribing medications as the first line of treatment and stepping up drug regimens when the first effort does not succeed. This jump to prescribe can also cause a cascade of complications as side effects from one medication can result in prescribing another medicine to deal with the side effects from the first prescription, and before you know it, the patient has multiple medicines interacting and causing symptoms that add to their suffering.

Advertising, marketing, and social media campaigns are partly responsible for the firestorm use of medications we are seeing now. After all, you can't turn on the TV or computer without being bombarded by pharmaceutical ads that promise a pill for diabetic nerve pain, a drug for rheumatoid arthritis, an anticoagulant that lowers the risk of blood clots and strokes, relief from headaches, abdominal distress, sore muscles, depression, even cancer, and so much more. Long gone are the days when famous jingles like Alka-Seltzer's popped into our minds for relatively minor every-day ailments like upset stomachs and headaches!

Did you know that the United States is one of only a handful of countries in the world that allow direct-to-consumer prescription drug ads?[2] It goes without saying that pharmaceutical companies are really taking advantage of this opportunity. You'll see them promoting TV commercials during popular shows such as dramas and news programs that their target audience is known to watch, usually the folks sixty-five and older who believe what they promise in the ads. They take out glossy full-page ads in magazines and put strategically placed pop-up messages on the Internet to attract people who suffer from a host of maladies, including depression, insomnia, and digestive issues that just about everyone experiences from time to time. According to recent research, TV ad spending by pharmaceutical companies has more than doubled in the past four years, making it the second-fastest-growing category on television during that time.[3]

Compounding this are the doctors who are featured guests on talk shows that promote certain pharmaceuticals. When he was a young doctor, Dr. Sinatra would be paid $1,000 by drug companies for giving a lecture on cholesterol, statins, and heart disease. "It was big money back then," he recalls, "But when I did research for them and sent in double blind studies, I was often shocked at what they did with the data."

It's no secret that drug companies pay doctors a substantial fee to promote their products, increasing the chance for medical mis-representation, which is becoming increasingly common these days. All his lecturing on cholesterol and heart disease came to a sudden and abrupt end when a peer-reviewed medical publication, approximately twenty-five years ago, revealed that statins, although excellent cholesterol killers, also blocked the same metabolic pathway of the production of Coenzyme Q10. CoQ10, in Dr. Sinatra's opinion, is the most important nutrient the body synthesizes. So, in short, some drugs can have some frightful, undesirable metabolic effects. That is not to say that all drugs are suspect. There are a lot of great products on the market today, but there are also a lot of ineffective ones as well, making it difficult for consumers to know who and what to trust.

Medical information is everywhere we look these days, but not all of it is accurate. It depends on who is doing the talking. Are you familiar with the comment that you can go to five different doctors and get five different opinions? Doctors are equally perplexed when it comes to the validity of the studies they depend on for their profession. It has been noted that roughly a third of the medical literature doctors read today in top-of-the-line medical journals has been declared fraudulent. Research is a big part of that misleading science because of the way it's conducted and calculated. Studies underwritten by pharmaceutical companies tend to report data based on relative rather than absolute risk. It's a difficult concept to understand. But when you are talking about relative risk, it is really only a fraction of what really occurs.

As Dr. Sinatra recalls, "For years and years, we doctors believed that cholesterol was the villain in heart disease until the Framingham Heart Study proved otherwise. When I was a young cardiology doctor, I participated in this decades-long study by sharing data. I remember towards the end of the study, doctors, who had preached that cholesterol was the enemy, were surprised to learn that they had been wrong in believing that people would die earlier with high cholesterol. That was a total paradigm shift for them and they had a difficult time accepting it. But the science showed them the facts. Up until that time, we doctors grew up with the notion that the higher the cholesterol, the fewer years a person would live. In other words, higher cholesterol predisposed them to strokes, heart attacks, dementia, and more. But now we know that cholesterol is vital for protecting neurons, and the workings of the brain among other things.

"What is constant is that medicine is always changing. I've seen that happen in my own lifetime when we treated gastric ulcers by surgically cutting them out and cauterizing them. Twenty years later it was discovered that gastric ulcers were caused by H Pylori, bacteria that could be successfully treated with antibiotics."

Many studies are refuted over time for many reasons. And that's not unusual. What is disturbing is that so many paid researchers embark on studies wanting certain end results and they capitalize on the ones, no matter how miniscule, that promise the effects they were hired to find. We tend to think of the scientific process as being objective, rigorous, and even ruthless in separating out what is true from what we want to be true, but in fact it's easy to manipulate results and arrive at conclusions you hope for, especially if there is money on the line.

Then there are those health proclamations that are publicized with authority and certainty, only to be walked back later as new developments and findings are discovered. These medical "never minds" tend to undermine our confidence and cause confusion. We saw it throughout the pandemic; we listened to changing recommendations and conflicting reports as we sought answers and sound guidance for the best and safest course of action to take to protect our health.

So what can we believe when we want to know what's best for our health, especially as we age?

Look at all of the studies that celebrate healthy lifestyles without promoting products. These studies take into account the choices people make in terms of their well-being, with no profit margin coercion influencing their findings. From unbiased research, ongoing clinical studies, and anecdotal observations, we know that we can improve our health by changing our habits and lifestyles, including eating organic foods, exercising every day, and avoiding harmful toxins in our diet and environment. In many cases, we can even reverse diseases naturally, without turning to prescribed medicines. People who have discovered the secret sauce to a healthier life have also added grounding to their daily routine.

Take a look at the health revelations of people who live in the so-called Blue Zones, the places where longevity and centenarians rule. The Blue Zones are areas of the world where people live one hundred years or more, with less stress, more connections, and fewer incidents of dementia and disease.[4] These regions include the Mediterranean, the Greek Island of Ikaria, Sardinia in Italy, Okinawa in Japan, Costa Rica's Nicola Peninsula, and Loma Linda in California. Common lifestyle factors among the residents include natural physical activity, such as walking or hiking and gardening. A large majority of the residents also grow their own fruits and vegetables in keeping with their preference for a fresh, seasonal diet.

Research shows that gardening can boost your mood and well-being while also providing a physical activity that's rewarding and productive.[5] Gardening is also one of the best ways to tap into the restorative powers of the Earth because you are putting your hands directly into the soil as you plant, weed, or harvest your vegetables. Similarly, because of the warm climates of the Blue Zones, people enjoy the outside all year round and do a lot of swimming, hiking, and walking, all common activities these communities share, and all great ways to get grounded if you are barefoot or wearing natural leather footwear while doing these outdoor activities. If people in the Blue Zones are still physically fit at one hundred years old, they must also have strong bones. Could it be that grounding helps with osteoporosis?

Researchers who have studied the longer-life phenomena of the Blue Zones attribute their longevity to their down-to-Earth lifestyle practices. We believe grounding has a lot to do with it. The breadth of validation from trustworthy data and real-life testimonials about grounding is absolutely enormous. As Hippocrates said, "Nature itself is the best physician." And with centuries-long evidence to support that heralded dogma, that is one piece of medical wisdom that you can count on.

For years, Sharon Whiteley was plagued by "white knuckle" circulation issues in her fingers and toes when the weather turned cold. After turning to her doctor for answers, she discovered she had Raynaud's disease. For most people, it isn't a disabling disease, but it can affect your quality of life. Doctors don't completely understand the cause of Raynaud's attacks nor can they suggest a cure, but they know blood vessels, especially in the hands and feet, appear to overreact to cold temperatures or stress. If Raynaud's is severe, reduced blood flow to your fingers or toes could cause tissue damage, gangrene, and more.

"While my doctor told me to avoid going outside in the cold weather and bundle up when I did, there was nothing more he could offer to help me with my winter woes. As I would later discover, the cure lay right at my feet, literally. Going outside for a morning walk guaranteed white fingertips and a numbing chill in my toes. Once I learned about grounding, my daily ritual changed, as did my susceptibility to the cold. Here's how I handle my Raynaud's now. I either sit barefoot on the ground when it's nice outside, or when the weather isn't cooperating, put on my grounding shoes and sit with my feet in direct contact with the Earth. After a short period of time, my white fingers tips come back to life with color and the numbness subsides. More often than not, when I come back inside, it looks like I just brushed my cheeks with blush, a benefit of the increased circulation from simply going outside and getting grounded. Raynaud's, like so many chronic conditions, is no match for Mother Nature."

When Step Sinatra was suffering through his life-threatening EMF poisoning, he saw countless doctors who remained as baffled about his deteriorating health as he was. They suggested countless medications to help with stress, diet, and physical ailments, trying different treatments during a number of hospital stays that never seemed to make a difference. Step continued his downward spiral until he was very close to death.

What ultimately helped him recover was his realization that whenever he was in direct, close contact with wireless technology that emits EMFs, like his cell phone or laptop, he reacted physically. For him the cure was basically as simple as stepping away from high-tech toxins and stepping back outside on the Earth, far from man-made interferences, to stay grounded. It took almost dying at eighty-seven pounds in the hospital to fully realize the effect that EMFs—and grounding—can have on the body. People who are strong and healthy may not notice EMF sensitivities at all, but for those as sensitive as Step, awareness can make all the difference.

Today you will find him living on an island in Greece, soaking in the sun's energy, breathing in the sea air, walking barefoot on the beach, working remotely, and disconnecting from devices that make him feel ill as often as possible. While technological achievements have made our lives easier, and medical advancements have most definitely increased our life span, it's the quality of our health that allows us to do the things we want and live our dreams and passions, he says.

"Look how many people are sick and constantly getting treatments. The merry-go-round of doctors, appointments, and therapies has become the norm in health care. Even when you consider the findings of researchers who study longevity in the Earth's 'Blue Zones,' they are missing one critical point. They believe that diet is mainly responsible for their long lives.[6] Indeed, it has some element of truth. What is important to note is that four out of the five Blue Zones are on coastal waters, including Costa Rica, Sardinia, Ikaria, and Okinawa, where grounding is at its best.

"I personally made it a travel agenda over the last fifteen years to go to all these places and figure it out for myself. In Okinawa, I remember the men in the taverns all walked barefoot. I thought that it was strange back then. And looking back on it, the floors were all stone, which I know now are naturally conducive to grounding. This stuck in my mind for years even before I learned about grounding.

"But the main point is this. In each Blue Zone, most of the people who live there are grounded significantly in a twenty-four-hour period. If you read the book, *The Blue Zones*, the authors write about gardening and 'hands in the dirt.' Well, if your hands are in the dirt, you're grounded! They found that gardening was a big part of life in each place. But the authors had no idea about grounding back then. And each one of these places has sea or ocean access, which means the locals are breathing in negative ions all day long and balancing their body's natural rhythm as they do.

"I realized this when I went to Ikaria this past year. The wind blows hard from the north consistently and sprays the entire inland with a rich blast of negative ions. Additionally, many of the older people I saw stayed in the sea for thirty to forty-five minutes at a time, soaking in the nutrients from the water. I see people doing this where I live on my island in Greece as well. It's incredible to see people in their eighties and nineties so active outdoors. I witness this almost daily. The lady who lives down the road from me gardens most every day and then goes for a ride on her donkey to get wild greens in the mountains. She is eighty-eight years old.

"It is my sheer observational theory that grounding promotes longevity. It's also quite obvious knowing what we NOW know. People in the Blue Zone areas are connecting with the Earth and one another each and every day. Cell phones and cell towers are rarely in sight, keeping these places relatively devoid of the technological pollution that can adversely impact their health."

Dr. Sinatra had a hip replacement twelve years ago and recently began experiencing severe pain when he walked. He has a metal rod in his hip and experiences hip inflammation now and then, but most of the time he walks just fine. He and his wife spend five months in Connecticut and seven months in Florida every year, enjoying both life in the woods and on the beach interacting with nature on a daily basis whenever they can.

When you are vacationing near a beach, lake, or river, you can benefit from grounding, too, by taking the opportunity to walk in the water—barefoot is best—to soak up the natural healing you can find underfoot. "When we are in Florida, I walk on the beach every day, usually right at the shore with the salt water lapping at my feet, grounding, with my fly rod in hand. Since I ground all the time, it alleviated any inflammation or pain I might otherwise experience from my hip surgery."

Walking barefoot on the beach enables you to take advantage of all the minerals that are found in the sand. Walking along the shoreline, or standing, with your feet buried in wet sand, adds even more beneficial effects for your body. It doesn't matter whether it is an outgoing or incoming tide, you just want to get the wetness of the sand on your feet. In fact, that is not only the essence of grounding, it's the pinnacle of grounding. Everything else goes below that. In other words, if you walk barefoot on the grass or concrete, or while you are wearing specially made grounding shoes, you'll still benefit from grounding. There are different levels. But *the* level, the #1 way to ground, is on wet sand on a mineral-enriched beach.

"They call our beach in Florida 'Shell Beach' because of all the washed-up shells that mix in the sand. Shells are loaded with minerals. When I am in Florida walking on the beach, I am getting all these minerals and grounding energy, and I have no difficulty walking at all. I walk like a champ despite the fact that my hip replacement is twelve years old," says Dr. Sinatra.

"In June, we return to our house in Connecticut. We don't live near the beach so I wear grounding shoes when I go for a walk.

Every morning, I make it a habit to head out for coffee at this little coffee shop that is only about 300 yards from my house. Last year, about two weeks after we arrived back in Connecticut, I started to have discomfort in my right ankle again. I remember saying to myself that it was getting harder and harder to walk. I didn't think about it at the time, but I realized that the pain starting happening after I left the seashore. It's amazing that when I walked along the beach, with my fly rod in hand, I could walk two miles without any discomfort at all. But when I got back to Connecticut, I had a complete reversal."

"The pain in my right ankle throbbed and the inflammation I had tamed in Florida came roaring back. Before I knew it, I was experiencing enormous pain in my foot, so I called my family practitioner. He referred me to a doctor of osteopathy who squeezed me into his schedule. During my appointment, he did an ultrasound on my foot and showed me that I had a lot of inflammation with a build-up of fluid in the joint space. He told me that he wanted to inject my right ankle with cortisone shots to help relieve my pain and inflammation. Even though I was hurting, I didn't waste a second before I responded with an emphatic no.

"I used to own thoroughbred racehorses. Because they tend to have a lot of trauma in their ankles from racing, we would inject them with cortisone shots to help relieve their pain and inflammation. I began to notice, after a few injections, many of the horses couldn't run anymore. Some couldn't even walk without limping. With those memories looming large, I told the doctor why I was opposed to his recommendation."

If you look at the whole inflammatory cascade, you wonder what is causing it. As we wrote earlier, inflammation is caused by many things, among them infection, trauma, EMF radiation, heavy metals, insecticides, pesticides, and the like. But the basis of grounding is that we get this plethora of electrons that floods the area of inflammation and basically reverses the whole inflammatory mechanism.

That's what happened in Dr. Sinatra's case. When he returned to Florida, he resumed his daily walks on the beach even though his ankle still caused him a great deal of pain. What happened next is the reason behind our steadfast belief in grounding.

"Once I started walking on the beach again, my pain literally evaporated. In a range of one to ten, with ten being the worst pain, it went from nine and a half down to a zero. It was incredible. A few weeks later, I started taking two-mile walks on the beach. That's when you know there's something really special about grounding. Today, in my role as a physician, author, and keynote speaker, I feel it is incumbent upon me to follow the oath I took in medical school, to do no harm and to share with future generations what I know. What people need to know is that we have an incredible healing resource right under our feet in grounding. It really is nature's miracle drug and it works."

As we have said throughout the book, grounding is the antidote for millions of people. And it's freely accessible to everyone no matter where they are.

We caution that grounding is not a cure for chronic diseases, but it often takes the pain away and relieves other symptoms that are a bane of these illnesses. It is our hope through this book, that grounding becomes the norm in people's everyday lives—their homes, workplaces, and when they are outside, basically everywhere they go in their daily routines.

We're not alone in our desire to help people live their best lives. Integrative doctors are turning to age-old treatments, like acupuncture and meditation, as part of an overall approach to health. With the rise in chronic disease and the associated pain syndromes that often go along with it, the medical community is taking note of how ancient practitioners saw the mind and body as connected and inseparable. Traditional medicine practices are built around the intangible ideas of wellness, vitality, and healing. Their prescription for treating illness incorporated ways to balance the body and unblock energy flow so the whole body could return to its natural state of equilibrium. Modern medicine, on the other hand, has typically placed more emphasis on acute illnesses and not on the idea of preventing the disease from taking hold in the first place. The goal should be to enhance and optimize the body's natural function, which is what grounding does.

Good medicine is based in good science. It is inquiry- and observation-driven and open to new paradigms that work in people's best interests. Grounding, while one of the Earth's oldest medical treatments, is also its newest in terms of today's modern-day practices. Continuing studies support its efficacy in reducing the inflammatory conditions that are making so many of us sick. Because it's free, you don't need a doctor's prescription to benefit from its healing properties, nor do you need insurance coverage to make it worth your while. All you need to do is take that first step and let Mother Nature do the rest.

9

ANIMAL WISDOM

When it comes to natural healing, animals have a sixth sense that leads them directly to what they need most. From birds and elephants to dolphins and dogs, animals, whether by instinct or learned behavior, have discovered ways to cope with parasites, pests, aches, and pains. This science of self-medication is called zoopharmacognosy (*zoo* for animal, *pharma* for drug and *cognosy* for knowledge).[1]

Wounded by a vicious attack, tigers have been known to dig holes deep in the dirt to receive healthful benefits from the Earth. Freed from snares that mangle and rip their limbs, wolves and foxes are known to retreat to earthen dens to allow nature to soothe their inflamed body parts. Injured animals, from elephants to monkeys, seek out nature's pharmaceuticals to soothe pain and initiate recovery. In addition to select botanicals, they include mud and clay baths, rich in healing minerals, as a topical skin treatment that helps fight disease-causing bacteria in wounds. Together with the anti-inflammatory effects of grounding, and the inherent medicinal remedies found in the Earth's surface, nature takes care of her own in wondrous ways.

While Dr. Sinatra was in medical school, one of his fraternity brothers contacted him about investing in one of his family's racehorses. "His father had recently passed away and my heartbroken friend had managed to sell six of his father's seven thoroughbreds. He hadn't been able to sell the remaining mare and asked me to help him out. Long story short, I ended up partnering with him, breeding his remaining mare, and producing a four-time winner right out of the gate. I was hooked and began breeding horses for the racing circuit. I even ended up getting my own farm in Maryland, where my horses thrived in the lush green pastures.

"A year later, my best friend was battling pancreatic cancer, while taking care of his own horses that were confined in the stable's paddocks on his small Long Island farm. Trying to lighten his work load, I had five of the horses transferred to my own farm in Maryland. Unfortunately, he hadn't been able to keep up with their care during the last year of his life and they were in sorry shape. Their bones were protruding beneath their emaciated flesh, open sores festered on their flanks and their once fiery spirits were extinguished in their desperate attempts to merely survive another day. Severely malnourished and infirm, a lack of exercise left many of them lame, along with other problems that affected their gastrointestinal, cardiovascular, and respiratory systems. Having been confined for such a long time, the horses' mental states were also compromised, leading to behavioral problems related to pent-up energy.

"In spite of their dire conditions, I packed them all up into a van and drove them to my own farm in Maryland where I planned to let them run wild in my sixty-acre field with my other healthy horses. My farm manager was against this, of course, cautioning me that the horses were so sick that they were going to die anyway. 'Keep in mind,' he reminded me, 'the odds are never in the horse's favor when dealing with a starving animal. Even with proper refeeding technique, about 20 percent of severely malnourished horses will die.'"

Daily exercise is also essential for the overall health of a horse. Not only does it increase the horse's stamina and endurance and strengthen ligaments and tendons in their legs, it improves the functioning of heart and lungs, aids in the motility of the digestive tract, improves the immune system, and increases their resistance to disease. "As far as I knew," notes Stephen, "these horses hadn't been exercised in months. My friend kept them in a stable the size of a postage stamp on property that was well under one acre. They really had no place to run, and with his illness, they were no longer being properly cared for. I told the vet I thought it best to let nature take its course here, not explaining that I had been learning all about the benefits of grounding at the time and was convinced the horses would not only survive on my farm, they would thrive."

"I assured him that the horses were going to love being out in the wild no matter what happened in the end. As long as they had access to water out there and extra hay to supplement the grass they could eat, they would be fine. 'Just wait and see,' I offered, 'no harm done.'

"Guess what. Not a single horse died. They were exposed to natural sunlight and grounding every day. They thrived like crazy, putting on hundreds of pounds of weight and racing through the fields without a care in the world. They became strong horses, like the ones I owned, testament to the power of grounding for all living beings. In other words, the animal world tells the truth. When given the opportunity to reconnect with the Earth's energy, these once sickly, broken-down horses, now forever wild, were the absolute picture of health."

Studies and clinical observations have found that our pets can suffer from the same degenerative conditions that affect us when we are disconnected from the Earth. Not surprisingly, dogs and cats in the wild tend not to suffer from those conditions, and one of the reasons why, in our opinion, is that all wild animals are naturally grounded because they live outside all the time.

The Sinatras have owned many dogs over the years but one of Steve's favorites was a chow chow named Chewie. She and he were attached at the hip. "We traveled everywhere together—including my office, where she never failed to bring smiles to my patients' and staff's faces, or to raise my spirit during long days. It broke my heart when she started having trouble getting into the car. But as it does for many dogs, getting around became hard for Chewie as she got older. Chewie was fourteen when we had to say goodbye. I still miss her dearly, and she's been an ongoing inspiration to me in my work to find the best ways to prevent and manage dog joint pain."

One of the worst things you can do for your dog's joint pain is to indulge his desire to just sit still. Low-impact exercise keeps joints moving, which helps restore and preserve both flexibility and strength, increase range of motion, improve blood flow to the tissue surrounding joints, and encourage a healthy weight. The only problem is that once joint pain sets in, your dog probably isn't going to be especially excited at the sight of a leash.

One way to address this is by changing up the type of exercise. If your dog likes swimming, the natural buoyancy of water makes it a safe, ideal environment for working out achy joints and muscles. Simply walking on the beach in wet sand and immersing in the salt water of the sea, both great ways to get grounded, help reduce inflammation in their joints.

Joint health is a "use it or lose it" proposition, so it's essential that you get out—whether it's around the neighborhood, the park, or even just the yard. Just stay mindful of your dog's limitations. Start out slowly with ten minutes once a day, until your dog works out the kinks. From there, you'll want to work up to twenty minutes or so once or twice a day, if you can.

Since time began, animals have lived in direct contact with the Earth. Their feet were always on the ground, they always breathed open air, and the sun and moon illuminated their days and nights, keeping their circadian rhythms in tune with nature. Even after their people moved into houses, most dogs remained outdoors. In the 1950s and 1960s, dogs were kept outside more often than they tend to be today and were still primarily functional, acting as a guard, children's playmate, or walking companion. Since the 1980s, there have been changes in the pet dog's role, such as the increased role of dogs in the emotional support of their owners. People and their dogs have become increasingly integrated in each other's lives. Now people and their pets are indoor creatures. Sure, dogs go for walks and enjoy other outdoor activities, but, like most of us, our dogs often spend more than twenty hours a day inside.

Fifty years ago, veterinarians were seeing animal patients primarily for acute injuries and infectious diseases, common for their outdoor lifestyles. Today, along with growing incidences of obesity from overfeeding and under exercising, pets are suffering from a host of chronic degenerative diseases including allergies and arthritis, just like we are. According to *Scientific American*, our family pets develop diabetes, heart disease, cancer, and more, just like humans do.[2] Skin conditions, stomach issues, and ear infections are the top three reasons dog owners bring their pets to the vet, and stomach issues, urinary tract infections, and skin conditions top the list for cat owners, according to Healthy Paws Pet Insurance's third annual *Cost of Pet Health Care 2018 report*.

What's at the bottom of these conditions? Inflammation. The common denominator in so many modern-day ailments, inflammation, goes rogue when we—and our pets—step away from nature's treatment table.

Take arthritis for example. The CDC estimates that about 23 percent of human adults have it, and the stats are similar for dogs.[3] According to the Arthritis Foundation, about 20 percent of dogs suffer from the disease, with a staggering 90 percent of older dogs presenting with painful arthritic joints in their later years. Veterinarians suggest that the incidence of arthritis in dogs is also correlated to obesity.

Overweight dogs have a much greater chance of developing joint disorders. Multiple studies have shown the link between being overweight and the increased risk and severity of arthritis.[4] This condition is particularly problematic for city dogs that don't have access to consistent outdoor exercise. Experts in dog behavior agree that too little exercise is causing epidemic levels of canine obesity, lethargy, and behavioral problems. According to the American Society for the Prevention of Cruelty to Animals, one in four dogs is now considered obese, and heart disease and diabetes are also on the rise.

"The lack of exercise can lead to arthritis or other orthopedic issues, chronic inflammatory diseases and even potentially cancer," agrees Marty Goldstein, DVM, author of *The Nature of Animal Healing* and *The Inside Spirit of Animal Healing* and one of the first integrative veterinarians in the industry.[5] "Exercise not only lifts depression but it boosts the immune system because the lymph system is activated by motion. The lymph system's nodes, vessels, and ducts are major players in the immune system, capable of filtering out and killing unwanted bacteria and organisms. Without movement, the lymph or body purification system stays in an almost dormant state.

"Work on the immune system and a body can start to heal itself and bring inflammation down. Support the immune system and amazing things happen. That's the secret to enabling the body to function and thrive, as nature intended. It works for people and animals," he says.

More and more veterinarians are practicing integrative medicine to support an animal's immune system, incorporating alternative modalities like energy healing to complement their treatments on their pet patients. Like us, they have found that energy healing work affects the emotional, mental, and physical bodies of the pets they treat. Working in tandem with the benefits of grounding, specially designed PEMF (Pulsed Electromagnetic Field) machines are now being used to ramp up the effects of healing electromagnetic energy, an invaluable life force. PEMFs simulate nature's grounding abilities by sending pulsed waves of low-level magnetic frequencies directly into the body. These therapeutic waves are uniquely able to pass through the skin to deeply penetrate muscle, bones, tendons, and organs to expedite recovery from the inside out. This powerful healing tool, which is good for muscle recovery, resetting the central nervous system, strengthening the immune system, and improving cellular health, provides the body with the energy it needs to repair itself. "PEMF therapy," states Dr. Goldstein is "the most effective mind-blowing therapy I have ever encountered in fifty years of using alternative modalities to integrate with conventional medicine." We think of this as grounding on steroids and more proof that grounding works wonders.

Just as we know that disruptions in the normal flow of energy eventually lead to physical illness and psychological symptoms in people, such symptoms are now commonly seen in indoor pets as well. Not only does staying indoors promote a sedentary lifestyle, which leads to the alarming rise in pet obesity, it disrupts their exposure to unfiltered natural light, which is needed by the hypothalamus and other glands for endocrine balance and optimum health. Veterinarians advise giving your pets access to natural light whenever possible by letting them stay outdoors or near an open window or on a screened porch so that nothing interferes with the full spectrum of natural light.

In *Health and Light: The Effects of Natural and Artificial Light on Man and Other Living Things*, author John Ott, a pioneer of time-lapse photography, discovered the vital role that natural light plays in the lives of plants and animals. Without it, plants can't set fruit, animals have reproductive problems, and humans and animals may develop a variety of modern illnesses.

Indoor lighting adds to the problem. Glass windows screen out ultraviolet light, which is a crucial part of the spectrum, but fluorescent and incandescent bulbs are incomplete in other ways. Any lights that change the appearance of colors can adversely affect the body. It's ironic that the fluorescent lights being touted for their energy efficiency may, according to light researchers, create a host of new health problems, while none of the bulbs labeled "full spectrum" include the complete spectrum of natural light. Of course, the blue lights from computer screens are another problem altogether when it comes to our health as we have discussed in Step's story and our chapter on EMF. In our homes, appliances and electronics can create localized EMFs that affect pets, but Wi-Fi floods indoor spaces with dangerous electrically charged particles that can adversely impact their health. We suggest that you limit your pets' EMF exposure by turning off your Wi-Fi at night, or by putting all of your devices on airplane mode to mitigate its effect on your indoor pet.

It goes without saying that modern building materials are also keeping our pets from being naturally grounded. When they are outside on the grass, walking in sand, on gravel, or even on concrete, their bodies are absorbing a constant flow of free electrons. When they're indoors, in our cars, or walking on asphalt, they are insulated from the Earth's energy flow.

If your pet spends most of the day and all of the night indoors, do what you can to increase his time outside. Resting or playing in a fenced yard is perfect, as are long walks, hikes, and swims. For pets not able to sleep on the ground, grounding pads provide contact with the Earth when they are indoors.

In addition to much-needed exercise for you and your pet, from horses to dogs and more, there is another benefit to interacting with your pet outdoors. Grounding pets transfer their healing energy to you simply through touch.

Horseback riding on dirt trails is grounding for both horse and rider wishing to tap into a power source historically honored. History attests that the Roman Empire produced some of the finest mounted warriors the world has known, yet they rode bareback. According to stories we heard, they believed that the "Earth spirit" rose up through the horse and into the body of the warriors, thus empowering them.[6]

If you have ever ridden bareback and felt the sweat of the horse on your skin, you may recall feeling a spark-filled connection to the horse that's unexpectedly charged with energy. That sensation embodies the transfer of charged impulses from horse to human, manifesting in a grounding sensation that actually comes from the Earth itself.

Like other prey animals, horses have a highly developed sense of energy perception. It is key to their survival. Today's environment is very different from that in which they were naturally created. Like us, they now live under constant bombardment from an invisible array of frequencies from cell phones, radio waves, and Wi-Fi signals. We ride them on artificial footing under LED lights and stable them on rubber mats.

Take them outside and let them interact with nature's healing resources without man-made interference and you'll find their health and happiness return in spades, like my horses' did.

It goes without saying: pets bring a lot to the table in terms of unconditional love, playing an important part in our lives.

Grounding helps heal all kinds of inflammatory ailments that your pet may suffer from and walking them is one of the easiest ways to ensure that they are accessing Earth's healing energy. As grounding enthusiasts, we love anything that encourages folks to walk on a regular basis. And we've never met a dog that doesn't want or need to be walked daily. Not coincidentally, research has shown that dog owners walk twenty-two minutes more a day than people without dogs. All those extra daily steps, pats, and hugs you take while grounding your dog can make a real difference in your health and well-being.

In their bestselling book, *The Forever Dog*, Karen Becker and Rodney Habib write, "Health travels up the leash. Humans don't necessarily like to exercise, we don't like to move our bodies—there are a lot of things we don't want to do for ourselves that we'll do for our dogs. The healthy strategies that we choose for our dogs can ultimately better impact and influence our own bodies because we're moving more, we're outside more. We're getting fresh air, we're getting some sun, we're interacting with people. And pretty amazing research shows that petting dogs helps reduce human cortisol levels. Just being around dogs can lower our heart rate and our blood pressure. So there are positive physical changes that occur when we look at dogs and when we pet dogs and when we play with dogs, especially outside. It's a mutually beneficial relationship."[7]

10

EMFs AND YOUR HEALTH

Hundreds gathered on New York City's Pearl Street one afternoon in September 1882 to watch an entire city block come to life, courtesy of Thomas Edison. With a flick of the switch, electricity surged through cables to provide businesses and homes throughout lower Manhattan with electric lights. People watching that day saw the future unfold faster than they deemed possible. Candles and gas lanterns were snuffed out in homes as light bulbs produced reliable light without the risk of fire. Factories and shops grew more productive and safer too with this new technology.

At the turn of the 20th century, electric power lines and indoor lighting spread across the world. Today, 90 percent of the world's population has access to electricity and uses electrical appliances.[1] That means lots of electricity and EMFs (electromagnetic fields) are created around the world.

What are EMFs? Simply stated, they are invisible areas of energy or radiation associated with the use of electrical power, both natural and man made. EMFs have been around since the birth of our universe and are present everywhere in our environment—the Earth, sun, and ionosphere are all natural sources of EMFs. Human-made sources of electromagnetic fields include electric power plants, appliances, microwaves, computers, cell phones, tablets, and more, each emitting unnatural frequencies that can throw our bodies' electrical systems off balance.

As we discussed earlier in this book, we are all electric beings. And we have our own magnetic fields. Our bodies function electrically. Our heart, lungs, and brains send electrical signals through our nervous systems to help us pump blood, breathe, and move, which means every single cell in our bodies is conductive. When we connect to the Earth's magnetic field, our bodies immediately get grounded to frequencies that are good for our health. As inventor and electrical engineer Nikolas Tesla wrote more than a century ago, "Our entire biological system, the brain and the Earth itself work on the same frequencies."

The Earth has its own unique heartbeat, known as the Schumann Resonance, with a natural frequency pulsation of 7.83 hertz on average. Since life began on our planet, every living being's biology has been attuned to this subtle field. In studying this phenomenon, scientists found that the Earth's fundamental frequency of 7.83 Hz is very close to that of human alpha wave rhythms.

These alpha waves are present in our brains during early sleep, deep relaxation, dreaming, and meditation. These waves help to regenerate cells and promote healing in our bodies and are proven to promote mental coordination, calmness, alertness, inner awareness, mind/body integration, and learning. Since alpha waves in our brain closely resemble the Schumann Resonance, these frequencies combined act as a form of "environmental synchronization." However, when the synchronicity is disrupted, our health can suffer.

Our planet's natural frequency emits negatively charged ions created in nature by the effects of water, air, and sunlight on the Earth's inherent electromagnetic field.

Because our bodies are primarily made of water and minerals, our bodies exist in a negative ionized state, making us very conductive.

For that reason, we function best when we are continually exposed to and in-tune with the natural frequencies of the Earth.

In contrast, technology like wireless mobile devices and Wi-Fi sources in our environment emit man-made electromagnetic fields, or EMF radiation. This can cause a variety of stress-related responses in the body. Not only does EMF exposure have thermal and biological impacts on our bodies, but also, electronic devices emit positively charged ions. High concentrations of positive ions—also known as oxidants or free radicals—from EMFs disrupt our bodies' natural frequency, which also can be detrimental to our health.

When we are in direct contact with the surface of the Earth, as we are when we are grounding, negatively charged ions transfer into our bodies, which can help neutralize the positively charged oxidants. This can help reduce inflammation and improve our overall feeling of wellness, which is why we recommend grounding every day to mitigate the effects of man-made EMFs.

These man-made electrical machines and devices create electromagnetic fields as part of their normal functioning. Electric fields are produced whether or not a device is turned on, whereas magnetic fields are produced only when current is flowing, which usually requires a device to be turned on. Power lines, on the other hand, produce magnetic fields continuously because current is always flowing through them. Electric fields are easily shielded or weakened by walls and other objects, whereas magnetic fields can pass through buildings, living things, and most other materials.

One hundred years ago, an eminent Austrian researcher by the name of Rudolf Steiner wrote about the dangers that man-made EMFs posed to humankind. Steiner was a man way ahead of his time, writing about issues that affected humanity and spirituality long before anyone else considered them. Of these were his prescient concerns about unnatural waves of electricity and radio frequency. He urged caution about this relatively new technology of the 1920s, telling people to beware of electricity and radio frequency, suggesting they may be harmful to our health. He cautioned, "Phenomena involving electricity and magnetism encompass a process on Earth or a sum of processes on Earth which are inwardly connected with what we must call both Earthly and non-Earthly. The field of electricity and magnetism is one which really ought to be studied more deeply in relation to human health and illness. The phenomena of electricity and magnetism have a close connection to what is intrinsically Earthly in nature."[2]

His fears turned out to be right on the mark. Now, one hundred years later, we are living in the toxic electromagnetic environment he warned about, where we are being bombarded by dirty electricity from advanced technologies—many of which are wireless—that can be detrimental to our physical, emotional, and mental health.

What's more, wireless technology is constantly evolving. Approximately every ten years, mobile companies release a new generation of wireless systems. Each generation is an upgraded, more advanced version of the last one. In 2019, 5G networks were released. The term "5G" stands for "fifth generation."

5G provides faster mobile communications. This is expected to support the increasing number of electronic devices and services, including self-driving cars, virtual reality appliances, telemedicine, surveillance, and more. This is in addition to the EMF-producing appliances and technology we use every day, from cell phones, Wi-Fi, and computers to microwave ovens, things we use all the time in our homes and businesses. 5G works by using higher frequencies on the electromagnetic spectrum. The frequencies range from 3.5 gigahertz (GHz) to several tens of GHz. Before 5G was launched, these higher frequencies weren't used in mobile networks. They were typically used in devices like security scanners.

Throughout the world, electrical systems are connected to Earth's surface and its negative charge to maintain stability and safety. These man-made electrical machines and devices create electromagnetic fields as part of their normal functioning. Electric fields are produced whether or not a device is turned on, whereas magnetic fields are produced only when current is flowing, which usually requires a device to be turned on. Power lines, on the other hand, produce magnetic fields continuously because current is always flowing through them. Electric fields are easily shielded or weakened by walls and other objects, whereas magnetic fields can pass through buildings, living things, and most other materials. The world's systems, from large grids and power stations to homes, buildings, and factories as well as the machinery and appliances that are operated by electricity, are thus, said to be grounded or Earthed. Herein lies the surprise. Research conducted for more than a decade has demonstrated that Earth's charge and storehouse of electrons represents a major natural resource of health and healing. Research on biological grounding is now suggesting that this very same electric charge on the planet's surface plays a governing and nurturing role for both the animal and plant kingdoms— a form of electric nutrition, so to speak. It appears to have the potential to restore, normalize, and stabilize the internal environment of the human body's countless bioelectrical systems that govern the functions of health and healing.

Throughout history, humans mostly walked barefoot and slept on the ground, or they used footwear and bedding fashioned from animal skins that became permeated with body perspiration or ground moisture and thus permitted transfer of Earth's electrons into the electrically conductive body. Through this mechanism, every part of the body could equalize with the electric potential of Earth.

Modern lifestyles, however, have increasingly created a barrier between humans and a natural conduction of Earth's electrons into the body. Since the 1950s, for example, humans have increasingly worn insulating rubber or plastic soled shoes, instead of traditional leather, fashioned from hides and largely conductive. Obviously, humans also no longer sleep in conductive contact with the ground as they did in times past.

The results of grounding research raise an important question. Does the current disconnect with Earth's electrons represent a critically important and overlooked contribution to physiological dysfunction and to the alarming global rise in inflammatory-related chronic diseases? The research, together with global anecdotal feedback, suggests that Earth's electric charge is fundamental for maintaining health and promoting healing.

On the other hand, EMFs produced by technology are increasingly seen as harming our bodies while ironically helping make our day-to-day lives easier. It is interesting to note that when 5G was being rolled out nationwide in the United States, airports across the country were clamoring for a pause, citing its potential interference with airplane radar systems.

But what about the potential effects it has on the human body?

The dangers of EMFs are unfortunately downplayed today, in part, we believe, because people have become so dependent on technology that they don't want to know of any potential problems with it. But it's time to acknowledge the truth. EMFs are almost like a biological weapon in that we can't see, taste, or feel them. Invisible, they are out there doing what could be irreparable damage to not only our health, but the health of future generations as well. Cellular technology damages the mitochondrial

DNA, the same mitochondrial DNA that is passed from generation to generation, from the grandmother to the mother to the daughter. There have been studies about how harmful cell towers and power plants can be, but for the large part, nobody is bringing it up. It has proven to be a controversial topic.

The technological age we live in brought us many amazing devices—microwave ovens, cell phones, and Wi-Fi connections, to name just a few. However, there appear to be serious EMF radiation health dangers associated with these tools of convenience. From unending work emails and hours spent scrolling through social media, to the constant barrage of non-stop media coverage, now more than ever before, we are overwhelmed by the constant distractions of technology.

Many chronic illnesses have risen in recent years, such as fibromyalgia, chronic fatigue syndrome, autism, and multiple sclerosis. The standard reasons given for the staggering rise—poor diet, lack of physical activity, and stress—hold true. However, there's another factor that's largely overlooked—the effect of electropollution on our bodies' operating systems. We are a nation hooked on technology. Not only do we depend on it, we expect it to be fast, reliable, and readily available. Nowhere is this more apparent than in the world of wireless technology.

Wireless technology allows us to communicate without the use of cables, wires, or some other physical medium. Remember back in the 1990s when you had to plug a cable into a wall to access the Internet? While you can still do that, most people have replaced this "archaic" practice with Wi-Fi (wireless fidelity), which uses radiofrequency signals to get us connected online.

Believe it or not, wireless technology is nothing new. In one form or another, it's been around since the early 1800s, starting with physicist Hans Christian Oersted, who established the relationship between electricity and magnetism—electromagnetics. Other physicists and scientists followed, including James Clerk Maxwell (who came up with Maxwell Equations) and Heinrich Hertz (who created radio waves and whose name to this day is used to is measure the frequency of radio transmissions . . . megahertz, gigahertz, etc.).

Without a physical medium guiding communication signals, the transmission of signals is accomplished with antennas, which turn electrical signals to radio signals in the form of electromagnetic waves. We've discussed the potential dangers of electromagnetic waves/radiation earlier in the book when we wrote about Step's story and his life-threatening electrosensitivity. But with advances in wireless technology, the health dangers of our exposure to chaotic vibrations are likely advancing as well.

All of this leads to unprecedented levels of radiofrequency radiation transmitted through homes and businesses and in the streets. In other words, people who live and/or work in cities or towns infiltrated with these cells will be in constant presence of this largely unstudied electropollution. Most government organizations and, not surprisingly, tech companies, advise that there is little-to-no reason to worry about potential health risks of EMFs.

But emerging research shows otherwise.

In 2011, the International Agency for Research on Cancer reviewed all the published literature to date on radiofrequency radiation and categorized it as a possible carcinogen.[3] Since that time, a broad range of adverse health effects have been associated with exposure. Some of them include schwannomas (tumors in the tissues that cover nerves), brain, and eye cancers, DNA damage, and infertility in men. Children are particularly at risk, as their thin skulls allow the brain to absorb more radiation than an adult brain.

In one rat study released in 2018 by the National Toxicology Program, researchers concluded that there is "clear evidence that male rats exposed to high levels of radio frequency radiation (RFR) like that used in 2G and 3G cell phones developed cancerous heart tumors . . . There was also some evidence of tumors in the brain and adrenal gland of exposed male rats."[4]

Another 2018 study had similar findings. Researchers noted a significant increase in heart tumors in rats exposed to the highest doses of radiofrequency radiation.[5]

The authors of a recent study on the rollout of 5G said it best: "Because this is the first generation to have cradle-to-grave life-span exposure to this level of man-made microwave (RF EMR) radiofrequencies, it will be years or decades before the true health consequences are known. Precaution in the roll out of this new technology is strongly indicated."[6]

5G is slowly but surely here to stay, and within the next few years, it will be hard to fully prevent exposure. But there are steps you can take to protect yourself, like grounding.

Grounding enables the energy of the Earth to flow directly into your body, bringing it back to your most natural electrical state and mitigating the effects of harmful EMFs. Do this every day, as the weather permits. Research has shown that when the body is grounded, "its electrical potential becomes equalized with the Earth's electrical potential through a transfer of electrons from the Earth to the body."[7] This helps lower radiofrequency radiation and 5G health concerns. And generally speaking, grounding keeps your metabolism and your capacity for healing and recuperation at maximum efficiency.

We are not advocating living without today's technology. After all, it has improved our lives in many positive ways. We are merely advising you to be mindful of the invisible threat it may pose to your health. Until definitive science shows that wireless technology is totally safe—which may not come for decades—we strongly recommending acting on the side of caution. It is our theory that current Wi-Fi frequencies are not congruent to the human biofield, but it is possible that in the near future, entrepreneurs and scientists will create Wi-Fi with harmonious ones.

A growing body of solid science points to concerning connections between electropollution and health. Studies suggest this fast-growing type of pollution can have very specific effects within our bodies and may lead to a wide variety of short-term and long-term health problems, even at levels of exposure well below current safety standards. Since 1990, there has been unprecedented growth of a variety of chronic diseases and conditions in the United States and beyond, including autoimmune, inflammatory, and neurological diseases; metabolic disorders; and chronic health conditions such as headaches/migraines, sleep disorders, fibromyalgia, and fatigue. Fertility issues, reproductive problems, and birth defects are also on the rise.

As its name suggests, dirty electricity is a form of electrical pollution. Also known as electromagnetic interference, line noise, or electrical noise, it refers to powerful, high-frequency electrical energy travelling on the wiring in buildings where only standard 50/60-Hertz AC electricity should be.

This type of electrical pollution is created by changes in the quality of electricity. Few modern electrical appliances and devices use standard AC electricity as is. Instead, they must manipulate standard electrical current to work, turning the flow of power on and off repeatedly, often thousands of times per second, causing very brief erratic changes in the voltage (known as "transients"). These changes can disturb the flow of standard AC electricity, creating irregular surges of electrical energy and unwanted higher frequencies—aka dirty electricity.

The erratic distortion of standard AC electricity creates unusable reactive energy. By travelling along wiring and power lines, this dirty electricity can radiate potentially hazardous electromagnetic fields (EMFs) into homes and workplaces.

As previously noted, symptoms of EMF exposure can include headaches, dizziness, insomnia, tinnitus, palpitations, and mood disturbances, and they can get much worse for those with increased sensitivities as you read in Step Sinatra's chapter earlier.

While it's nearly impossible to avoid EMF exposure completely, there are practical ways to limit it. Given the number of EMFs that bombard you all day long, getting educated about the negative effects of EMFs is imperative. If you are dealing with a serious illness, it is well worth your time to reduce your EMF exposure as much as possible. If you have been told EMFs are safe and not a danger to humans, I urge you to reconsider.

It is important to note that not all EMFs are bad. Sunlight and UVB that make vitamin D in your skin along with near-infrared radiation (IR) are very healthy EMF frequencies that we need regular exposure to if we hope to optimize our health. Broadly speaking, EMFs are categorized into ionizing and nonionizing radiation. Most agree on the hazards associated with ionizing radiation, which is why the dental hygienist covers you with a lead apron when taking X-rays. Similarly, you would expect to get sunburned if your bare skin was overexposed to the sun's powerful UV rays, which is a form of ionizing radiation. Ionizing radiation is generally believed to have enough energy to break the covalent bonds in DNA, but actually most of the damage is due to the oxidative stress resulting in excessive free radicals. Non-ionizing radiation is a type of low-energy radiation that does not have enough energy to remove an electron (negative particle) from an atom or molecule. Non-ionizing radiation includes visible, infrared, and ultraviolet light; microwaves; radio waves; and radiofrequency energy from cell phones.

What can you do to mitigate your exposure to bad EMFs?

Shut off the electricity to your bedroom at night. This typically works to reduce electrical fields from the wires in your wall unless there is an adjoining room next to your bedroom.

When using your cellphone, use the speakerphone and hold the phone at least three feet away from you. Seek to radically decrease your time on the cell phone. When you are not using it, put it in airplane or flight mode. While you may think the majority of your radiation exposure comes from outside your home, most of it is very likely coming from the items inside your home and the homes of your closest neighbors.

Again, we would like to stress that electropollution from Wi-Fi and other sources can be especially problematic for children because they don't have defense mechanisms to fight the effects of this constant threat. In fact, kids tend to be more vulnerable to Wi-Fi health effects and other electropollution than adults because they're smaller, their skulls are thinner, and their brain tissues are far more absorbent. Research shows that children's brains absorb twice as much electromagnetic radiation as adult brains. Even unborn babies are prone to Wi-Fi dangers in utero. A Yale study using mice showed that fetuses exposed to electromagnetic radiation were more hyperactive and had impaired memory due to altered neuron development.[8] And a study out of Korea that followed a group of seven- and eight-year-olds for five years found that those who used their cell phones for three or more minutes a day had a higher risk of ADHD (attention-deficit/hyperactivity disorder).[9]

Exposure to EMFs is not a new phenomenon for living beings. All living beings have always been exposed to natural electromagnetic fields, but the growing impact of technology-made EMFs on humans and the world we live in is creating more questions than answers.

The bottom-line problem is that *we just don't know all the answers yet.*

What we do know is that the Earth's electromagnetic field can empower us to take charge of our own health and mitigate the ill effects of dirty electricity, every day. We recommend grounding for at least an hour a day to keep the ill effects of EMFs away by keeping your blood flowing, lowering inflammation, and resetting your body's natural balance with the following caveats:

The strongest electric fields can be found beneath high-voltage transmission lines, so avoid grounding and walking in areas with extensive power lines. Transformers reduce this high voltage before it goes into your home or business, with the building's walls shielding you to some degree. But directly beneath the power lines is where the field is strongest. Both fields (electric and magnetic) drop off significantly with distance. The further you are from high-voltage power lines, the weaker the field and the safer you are. Be cognizant of staying away from areas where radio and cell towers are too, keeping a safe distance from them at all times.

Leave your cell phones at home when you are grounding outside. If you must bring it with you, carry it in a bag that blocks radiation and use the speaker function when taking calls. This will reduce RF exposure to your head. Some earpieces do generate and emit fields, but not nearly as much as your phone. By using earpieces or speakerphone, you can greatly reduce exposure to your head. If you do use an earpiece, make sure there is a hollow tube with the apparatus, as wires alone may conduct EMFs in to the sensitive ear tissues.

When you go back inside, keep your distance from appliances too as the EMF strength around appliances diminishes rapidly with distance. Don't sit or linger near appliances. You need to get up close to turn on the television, open the fridge or microwave, and load the washing machine. Just keep these close encounters short.

We spoke about EMF exposure with an integrative doctor who became interested in the health effects of non-ionizing radiation after she was given a cell phone that caused her middle finger to burn with neuropathic pain.

Researching medical journals on the health effects of wireless exposure, she was shocked to see decades of solid evidence linking "diseases of civilization" with exposure to man-made EMFs, yet there was a total disconnect between the published science, medical education, and clinical practice. Replacing the cell phone she was given with one that emitted lower radiation resolved her painful finger and she used it without further issues.

But her interest was piqued. She left the university and opened her own integrative internal medicine practice where she saw a growing number of patients with chronic fatigue, autoimmunity, neuropsychiatric conditions, and diabetes who continued to deteriorate despite optimal medical therapy. Her research and anecdotal cases with her own patients, coupled with clinical studies from various medical authorities, confirm that wireless radiation is a scientifically proven environmental toxin. Like us, she believes grounding is a good broad-spectrum health promotion that can help protect your health.

People don't realize that there are EMFs in their own homes; everyday appliances, like washers and dryers, emit harmful waves of electricity. Dr. Sinatra relies on a RAD meter to measure the EMFs in the rooms he frequents including the hotel rooms he stays in while traveling.

"The technology is incredible. RAD Meters—portable hand-held, electronic instruments used to detect radiation—give you an actual visual picture of the voltage you come in contact with. My own personal experience using these meters has demonstrated an incredible amount of EMFs that most of us aren't even aware of in places we thought were safe. Anecdotal studies have found that 5 percent of the world's population, my son included, can feel toxic EMF and it literally makes them sick. People are getting such bizarre illnesses today. And it doesn't just affect one of our body's systems. It affects their neurological system, their endocrinology, the brain and their reproductive systems. Some of our body's endocrine organs, like the thyroid, are very sensitive to EMFs. There's so much hypothyroidism in our country right now because of cordless and cellular phones and the like and no one has talked about the link between the technology and the disease. Here's the bottom line. If you have multi-systemic illnesses, neu-rological, endocrinological, and immunological at the same time, it could be from EMFs.

"It is overwhelming for doctors, because their patients are increasingly coming in with all these crazy symptoms. 'I can't sleep. I've got digestive problems. I'm dizzy. I have non-stop headaches. My body tingles all the time. I'm getting sore throats. I'm getting this, I'm getting that' and the doctors don't know what's causing their conditions and become overwhelmed. But if a doctor can't figure it out, I can tell you from years of experience, it's one of three things. Either they have undiagnosed Lyme disease, exposure to black mold, or they have EMF poisoning. They can't see, taste, or feel these toxic vibrations, but it's frequently a combination of all three. And that's why these people are so sick. That's what happened in Step's case and basically grounding saved his life."

This book is about protecting your own body, being your own detective, your own doctor, your own healer. One of the pearls of this book is to enlighten you about healing your own body, and it's a very simple way to do it. You avoid things that are bad for your body and do things that are good for it.

We've said it before. We live in a soup of toxins, from pollution to dirty electricity, that is affecting our health. But nothing trumps Earth's energy to get it back on track again. Take a day off from electronics, or even several days, and detox from toxic technology. You may not be a canary in the coal mine like Step is, but all those new aches and anxieties you may be feeling just might be telling you to get grounded and get your health back! Your body will thank you!

Scientific studies, many of which are listed at the back of this book, show links between chronic EMF exposure and a variety of health problems. If you have one or more of these conditions, consider the source and unplug from technology as often as possible.

- Cancer
- Diabetes
- Chest pain or pressure
- Heart palpitations and arrhythmias
- Asthma
- Infertility
- ADD/ADHD
- Behavior/learning problems

- Concentration issues
- Memory problems
- Depression
- Anxiety and irritability
- Sleep disturbances
- Headaches
- Muscle and joint pain
- Leg and foot pain
- Fatigue and weakness
- Numbness and tingling sensations
- Itching and burning sensations
- Facial flushing
- Tremors and muscle spasms
- Sinus problems
- Digestive issues

To give yourself the most protection from EMF radiation:

Use a Corded Landline: For most phone calls I make or receive, I'm content to wait for a landline. Cordless phones, which have become the norm in most households, generate alarmingly large amounts of EMF radiation compared to phones with cords.

Change Computer Connections: Hardwire your computers to an ethernet connection to avoid exposure to WiFi.

Only Use Cell Phones on Speaker: Never put a cell phone up to your ear and near your brain. Instead, put it on speaker and move the phone away from your body. Plus, you never—let me repeat never—want to give a cell phone to a child because their bodies are even more susceptible to the radiation.

Find a Place to Carry Your Cell Phone: Never carry your cell phone on your body, such as in breast pockets, pants pockets, or in bras. Researchers have identified clusters of breast nodules in the shape of a cell phone among those who stashed their phones in their bras. Stow your phone in a carrying bag.

Know the SAR: When purchasing a cell phone, find out its specific absorption rate (SAR). SAR is a way of measuring the quantity of radio frequency energy that is absorbed by the body. The lower the SAR of a cell phone, the better it is. I wouldn't consider any cell phone model with a SAR level of more than 0.5.

Avoid Microwave Ovens: Not only do microwave ovens emit EMFs, they break down vitamin B12 in your food into inactive substances, release potentially toxic compounds from food packaging, and cause a loss of antioxidant compounds in vegetables. Instead of microwaving your food, cook it on the stovetop or in your oven.

Become an EMF Detective: Consider buying an electropollution detector. Electropollution detectors can tell you how strong EMF radiation waves are—and how far they extend beyond their source.

11

EVERYDAY GROUNDING

Getting started with grounding is easy. If conditions allow, all you have to do is literally go barefoot outside. Just twenty to thirty minutes a day can make a difference in your health. More, of course, is even better. You can never overdo it.

If going barefoot outside isn't realistic, a warm basement with a concrete floor will also work. Sit there and read or just relax with your bare feet or grounding footwear (shoes or socks) touching the ground. Ground every day for just this limited period and see how it affects your pain or stress level. Sit, stand, or walk on grass, sand, soil, unsealed tiles, or concrete—even better if it's damp for greater conduction of the Earth's electrons into your body. These are all conductive surfaces from which your body can draw the Earth's electrons. Carpets, wood, asphalt, plastic, rubber, and vinyl are not conductive.

Ideally, you want to sustain the grounding experience and make it a part of your daily routine to access all of its health benefits. And do it consistently. Like filling up your gas tank, grounding needs to be replenished. It is not cumulative. Ever since we learned about grounding, we each found different ways to connect to the Earth depending on where we are. Step calls a Greek island home and follows in the footsteps of ancient Greek healers and athletes who declared that nature is the best physician, along with practicing Qigong daily. Sharon thrives in the sunshine and dry climate of Arizona, renowned for heart-healthy lifestyles. Dr. Sinatra lives for the time he spends on his favorite Florida beach and the incomparable healing he receives from grounding and fly fishing in the surf. The beauty of grounding is that you can do it anywhere and everywhere in every climate and environment and its feel-good effects are virtually instantaneous. You'll not only be keeping your body in balance naturally, you'll be addressing a host of inflammation-related ailments while you are it.

We've put together a helpful grounding guide to get you started on the path to good health; however, it's been our experience that once people start to reconnect to the Earth, they find their own way to make it an integral part of their lives.

Remember the story about the bush bartender in the Bahamas we spoke about earlier in this book? She learned about healing techniques from her ancestors and knew how to heal people with herbs and botanicals that grew wild. She related a fantastic story about using the outgoing tide as a way of healing the body and detoxing the lymph system. The lymph system of the body harvests all our toxins. Stated simply, if we keep the lymph flow going, toxins won't get stuck in our body; we naturally discharge them by doing things like moving and sweating, both of which help to detoxify the body.

One of the best ways to dislodge and eliminate toxic sludge is by rebounding on a trampoline. A few minutes a day will expel poisons by jostling the lymph nodes and squeezing the toxins out. A lot of the toxins we are exposed to enter our bodies and lie just beneath the surface of the skin, including mercury, insecticides, and pesticides. You can also sweat out these chemicals in an infrared sauna or do Ayurvedic skin brushing; commonly known as dry brushing, this practice involves a stimulating lymphatic massage to detoxify the lymphatic system, refresh your skin, and revive the mind. There are certain herbal choices and maneuvers you can use to help detoxify your body as well, including the arm movements that conductors have perfected.

What conductors do as they lead orchestras is really a type of Tai Chi, an ancient Chinese tradition that keeps the body in constant motion through gentle low-impact exercise and stretching. People practice Tai Chi for a number of reasons, including to reduce stress, anxiety, and depression, to improve their mood and aerobic capacity, and to increase their energy and stamina. Tai Chi also enhances the immune system and discharges toxins. The fact that there are more classical music conductors who live to be one hundred than any other profession speaks volumes about the importance of moving and constantly detoxifying the body.

On his Qigong journey, Step met a Buddhist monk who shared the same insights about the importance of moving and swinging your arms to mobilize your body fluids, and now Dr. Sinatra swings his arms as he walks along the shore of his beach in Florida, grounding as he goes.

"The bush woman reminded me about the role the outgoing tide plays in helping detoxify your body. Now I also swing my arms as I walk in the surf, doubling the detoxification process. If you stand in the surf when the tide is strong, and you dig your heels into the sand to avoid being knocked down or washed out to sea, the water pulls hard against your feet. When the tide pulls against the body and gravity brings down the blood as you are standing, the body is being discharged of toxins. As a scientist, it makes a lot of sense to me for many reasons, not the least of which is its connection to grounding and the detoxifying effect it has on our body," says Dr. Sinatra.

As you know, we need detoxification more than ever. We live in a soup of EMF, computers, Wi-Fi, cordless phones, cellular phones, and cell towers, and this electromagnetic energy is destroying our DNA. We exist in a sea of chemicals with GMOs and processed foods. Our environment is not only prone to all manner of deadly viruses, but also pollution in our air, water, land, and soil, not to mention noise and EMF pollution, is also threatening our well-being.

How do you protect yourself? It's as easy as getting back to nature and getting back to basics. Do the things that make sense, that won't compromise you and don't cost anything. Grounding is not only the best way to start, it's life-saving and it's free. If you knew you could reduce joint pain simply by walking on the grass or the beach, wouldn't you consider grounding right now? While grounding might not put an end to all your ailments, it can definitely reduce the pain and stiffness caused by inflammation that impact your day. Some people experience a tingling or a blush on their cheeks as they ground and others don't feel any sensation at all. Grounding is a very subtle energy. You won't feel a jolt.

There are many different ways to get grounded, even when you can't get outside. All it takes is direct contact with the Schumann energy of the Earth and you are on your way.

When the weather is nice and you live in a city, head outside to a park, a garden, a patch of grass, or even a solitary tree whose roots run deep into the Earth. Any place that you can actually touch the unpaved ground works for grounding. Make tracks for the nearest plot of land; anywhere trees, plants and grass grow is ultimately where you want to go. Season permitting, kick off your shoes, and plant your feet on the ground—even a mere ten minutes will do. Lean against a tree, and your circulation will rev up within minutes even if you feel no sensation. Holding onto a leafy branch or tree limb will ground you too, especially if your hands are damp.

Sitting on the Earth, or on a cloth or blanket made of natural loosely woven fibers, does wonders for what ails you. In ancient yoga texts, they talk about the gurus sitting on animal skins, which are naturally conductive when placed directly on the ground, grounding as they practiced their healing arts. If you have an arthritic hip or sore knee, try to position that painful spot so that it's touching the ground. Even better, lie down for a spell, letting your entire body stay in close contact with the Earth, and feel your stress melt away. Like the bottoms of your feet, your skin absorbs electrons, helping reduce chronic inflammation and the discomfort it causes, including tension headaches, backaches, and more.

If nature is nowhere near your home, put on grounding footwear—they are specially made to let you ground while you walk, even on concrete city sidewalks. Unlike the asphalt used on streets, concrete is a conductive surface that enables the energy to flow between you and the Earth. Concrete is simply reconstituted sand and water and it allows for the transfers of electrons. Don't shy away from a stroll in the rain either. Drizzles can be beneficial as conductivity is enhanced by moisture. Sealed surfaces, such as glazed tiles, along with vinyl, carpeted, and wood floors are insulators and they don't allow electrons in. And because roadway asphalt is fabricated from petrochemicals, it's out, too.

Footwear with technically crafted conductive soles provides grounding. Because the soles of most shoes are made from synthetic materials, you won't be able to receive the health benefits of grounding while you are wearing them. Why is this important? Because your feet have the most nerve endings per square inch of skin than any other part of your body.

Among the five meridians in the human body that guide energy throughout, the Chinese identified a major energy point on our feet some three thousand years ago. According to studies by leading acupuncturists at the Modern Institute of Reflexology, it is believed that the K-1 (kidney) Meridian point, the only meridian origin on the bottom of the feet, holds a reputation for dramatic healing response.[1] Today you can find grounding footwear that is engineered to ground the KI point of the foot—also called the metatarsal area or ball of the foot just below the big toe—enabling the wearer to benefit from the most direct energy flow while wearing the shoes outside.

If you practice yoga or Tai Chi, you may not be aware that these mind and body exercises have been historically and traditionally done in bare feet. The central focus involves "growing a root" that allows for the opening of a pathway between the Earth and the body by way of the feet. Certain yoga poses also employ a sense of grounding, allowing your body and mind the opportunity to release anxieties and physically join you to the Earth. With yoga as a grounding mechanism, you rely on both your mental focus and connection to the Earth in order to experience a balance of the mind and body.

Guided meditation can also help to align your energies with the Earth's energies so that you feel calm, refreshed, and at peace. There are many meditations that are used in grounding, some are performed inside; others are practiced outdoors, sitting on the ground or perched against a tree. Plants and trees have their own energy fields and you can absorb this energy in a positive and revitalizing way for your whole being.

If you can't go outside, think metal and flowing water, touching both can keep you grounded. Add salt to your bath water in a porcelain tub and in the shower, place your hand on the shower head and your feet on the metal drain to take advantage of its grounding properties while the water is running. Water passing from the ground through the metal pipes transfers electrons with every drop. You can also hold onto the bathroom or kitchen sink faucet while the water is running to access grounded energy from the Earth. Do you have a fireplace in your house? Place your hands directly on the stone and keep them there for ten minutes or more.

When weather or the dark of night keeps Dr. Sinatra inside, he takes a short walk on his bathroom floor, custom designed and fabricated with concrete and built to enable him to ground whenever his bare feet touch the surface. You don't need to go to that extreme to make your home a grounded sanctuary. There are products you can purchase that bring the power of nature inside, including grounding sheets that promise a better night's sleep.

Where you live can be a hot bed of technology, emitting a constant flood of radiation from electromagnetic fields, cell phones, computers, and Wi-Fi—all of which assault your body and contribute to free radical stress. Grounding helps ameliorate your exposure to the harmful effects of modern-day communications, not to mention the onslaught of harmful pollution from car exhaust, cigarette smoke, fertilizers, insecticides, and more, and is critical to buffering the effects from the trappings of modern life.

Along with making it a habit to ground each day, disconnect from your cell phone, your iPad, and any other wireless device that relies on man-made electromagnetic fields to get powered up as often as you can and especially in your bedroom at night when you are a sitting duck for unseen sensory overload.

Country dwellers live in grounding nirvana. A growing body of research shows that people who spend time outside in sunny, green, and natural spaces are happier and healthier than those who don't. Fascinating scientific studies by Japanese researchers interested in finding out what happens when people spend time in nature showed measurable beneficial changes in the body, including lowering the stress hormone cortisol and inducing a state of physiologic relaxation. They noted that when people walk through forests, as they do in a practice the Japanese call "forest bathing," they often exhibit changes in the blood that are associated with protection against cancer, better immunity, and lower blood pressure. Recent studies have also linked nature to symptom relief for health issues like heart disease, depression, cancer, anxiety, and attention disorders. It is no surprise that grounding supercharges these findings.

We noted that the long-living residents of the "Blue Zones" are avid gardeners. The sensory experience of gardening—literally putting your hands in the dirt, digging, and helping something grow—actively fosters a sense of calm satisfaction, eases stress, and improves your mood and focus. A study conducted in Norway concluded that people who were suffering from depression and who spent six hours a week for three months growing flowers and vegetables experienced a measurable improvement in their depression symptoms.

Other research suggests that the combination of physical and mental activity involved in gardening is not only therapeutic, it lowers the risk of developing dementia. You've heard of memory gardens? Residential facilities have found that Alzheimer's patients can walk through them without getting lost. The sights and smells of the gardens alone promote relaxation.

Many urban areas have introduced community gardens for their residents, so consider becoming involved to get grounded while you are growing those healthy vegetables and herbs.

Spending time in the garden is great for nurturing your own well-being, too.

Do you live near a botanical garden? We can't imagine a better place for grounding. There are some 1,500-plus gardens across the globe, each a bouquet of science and delight, making folks aware of both the beauty and the bounty of nature. Some gardens hold classes in Tai Chi, Qigong, meditation, yoga, Pilates, even swing dancing, along their garden paths—perfect pairings for life-altering grounding opportunities.

Since salt water is a great energy conductor and sand, mineral rich, is equally so, the benefits of spending time at the beach are indisputable. Whether you spend a week at the beach for your long-awaited vacation or you are one of the privileged who live near it year-round, it is a wellspring of healing properties. The moment you step on the beach and take in the salty sea air, you breathe easier. For centuries people looked at the sand and surf as a fully stocked pharmacy. We bask in its ability to heal cuts and skin ailments, reduce inflammation, soothe the soul, and restore energy. Oceans aside, mountain streams, river bends, ponds, and lakefronts also offer up electron-nourishing strolls or dips, so if you have the opportunity, take off your shoes and walk in the water whenever you can.

Loss of sleep can trigger tissue-damaging inflammation according to new research. Studies show that grounding during sleep has the ability to reduce a person's nighttime cortisol levels, resynching them with the Earth's natural twenty-four-hour circadian cycle and restoring natural sleep patterns. Not only can you sleep better and wake refreshed, you can keep fatigue, pain, and emotional stress at bay. People who sleep grounded say that their daytime energy levels increase as their nighttime pain levels decrease.

Because weather and whereabouts can limit our access to nature, commercially manufactured devices that connect to the energy of the Earth, via the grounding port in electrical outlets, are becoming even more readily available. These indoor-use products are designed to promote conductivity of the natural electron flow while we are sleeping, engaging in exercise, or taking part in indoor activities. There are even conductive grounding pads for connecting your body to the Earth while you're sitting at your desk at work and grounded sheets that promise you a restorative night in bed.

Step Sinatra, whose ultra-sensitivity to EMFs has sent him to the far corners of the Earth to find safe zones, has a few grounding secrets while he is traveling.

"Today's computerized cars can expose you to a lot of radio-active frequencies while you are driving. And if you use your cell phone, it gets even worse as the signals can be up to five times stronger than the ones you normally connect to when you are not on the move. I make a point to get out of the car as often as I can to get grounded. I either put my hands or feet directly on the ground or I grab onto a guard rail and hold it for a few minutes. Guard rails are made of steel and are always grounded so I can get grounded too. When I arrive in my hotel room, I bring a continuity tester with me to verify if and how well things are grounded in the room. The steel lights that are often found next to the beds are grounded, as are window sills and occasionally door knobs. Simply touching these items assures that I am getting grounded while I am in contact with them."

You may not have thought about why aging musicians like the Rolling Stones still have the energy to perform their amazing live concerts, but we think it has a lot to do with grounding. As Step recalls when he played the electric guitar, "musicians are getting grounded the entire time they are playing their music, often up to five or six hours in a single day. The strings are made of steel and the instrument is plugged into a grounded amplifier giving them added boosts of grounding whenever they strum." Could grounding be the secret fountain of youth?

Still on the fence about grounding for your daily health regimen? Take a look at the everyday ailments so many of us suffer from, and you might find common ground with this alternative health resource.

If you feel tired all the time, you may have a problem with inflammation that you are not aware of. Medical researchers agree that fatigue remedies that address inflammation are key to getting your energy back. These include natural and lifestyle therapies involving nutrition, stress reduction techniques, exercise, lifestyle changes, and grounding.

How about allergies? Lifestyle and dietary modifications are now thought to be great first steps in treating allergies. The easiest step to take to keep allergies in check is to go outdoors and get grounded. The overall reduction of inflammation in your body after just ten to twenty minutes of direct contact with the ground can reduce or almost eliminate your nasal congestion and inflammation, and is an important way to combat your seasonal allergies.

Ailing with arthritis? Scientific studies have shown that physical activity, like walking and swimming, decreases the pain of arthritis and improves function, mood, and quality of life for its sufferers. Regular exercise can help with weight loss, too, not only lessening the strain placed on inflamed joints, but actually decreasing the progression of the disease. To keep arthritis symptoms in check, many doctors suggest walking or swimming for at least 150 minutes per week, both of which are key grounding activities.

Have an aching back? Back pain is one of the most common reasons for medical attention in the United States, with problems often found in the muscles, tendons, bones, ligaments, discs, or an underlying organ like the kidneys.[2] Aches and pains in the lower back can be chronic and are often caused by inflammatory arthritis, rheumatism, bone disease, or curvature of the spine. No matter where, when, or how it starts, back pain affects sleep, mobility, and mood. It may seem counterintuitive to consider taking a walk outside when even the slightest movement can manifest in breathtaking pain. If exercise is too much to fathom when you are in pain, simply lie down grounded to the Earth or sleep grounded.

We mentioned earlier that diabetes is becoming increasingly common. Managing diabetes is a challenge every day, and keeping blood sugar levels in the desired range is a constant balancing act. The good news is that diabetes can be prevented and controlled by lifestyle choices that include diet, exercise, and stress management practices like yoga, meditation, guided imagery—and grounding. As Dr. Stephen Sinatra pointed out in "New Hope for Diabetes," an article he authored, "our experience and observations over a fifteen-year period clearly indicate that grounding indeed holds great promise as a preventative and therapeutic strategy."

Worried about your heart? Dr. Sinatra participated in a grounding study on blood thickening, or viscosity, published in *The Journal of Alternative and Complementary Medicine*, entitled "Earthing (Grounding) the Human Body Reduces Blood Viscosity—A Major Factor in Cardiovascular Disease." The conclusions offer validating proof: "Grounding increases the surface charge on red blood cells and thereby reduces blood viscosity and clumping. Grounding appears to be one of the simplest and yet most profound interventions for helping reduce cardiovascular risk and cardiovascular events."

Given grounding's ability to reduce blood viscosity (that is, make blood thinner), it's best to be cautious when grounding at first if you're taking any medication related to blood viscosity, especially Coumadin (warfarin). This potent blood thinner is widely prescribed to patients with cardiovascular conditions that raise their risk for blood clots. People on Coumadin should also be cautious when considering whether to sleep grounded.

We suggest taking it slowly when you first try grounding; start with simply walking barefoot in the backyard, on the beach, or at the park. Or, try using a grounding device inside your home for an hour or two while relaxing or reading a book. Sleeping grounded should be considered only after you have gradually increased your grounding activities and have closely monitored its effects on your blood thickness. If you do prefer to sleep grounded for several hours or more while taking a Coumadin-like blood thinner, you must work closely with your physician as the combination of long grounding and potent blood thinners can make your blood too thin, resulting in possible bleeding. We can't emphasize enough that you must be cautious if you are taking potent blood thinners.

Although we say grounding is easy to do wherever you are, there are certain other caveats we would like to bring to your attention. For example, stay away from tall grass where Lyme disease–carrying deer ticks are found and avoid walking near electric power stations and cell towers, purveyors of dirty electricity. Barefoot walking can be dangerous too with sharp stones, sticks, broken glass, and other litter underfoot, so put on footwear with conductive soles to protect your feet. Don't walk the dog any place that could be harmful either.

We advocate safety when out and about, which is why you may want to consider wearing leather-soled footwear or purchasing grounding shoes for those long walks outside. If you are allergic to bees, don't picnic in the grass where you might get stung, and always be wary of any animal that may be lurking in the woods just off the trail you are following. Make sure the running faucet you are holding is not too hot to touch and that the guard rail you may grab is well off the road. In other words, you want to be productive not self-destructive when you are grounding for your health.

Find a place to ground that's free from cars and pollution too so you can breathe in clear air while you take in Earth's nourishment. Avoid grass sprayed with pesticides as they will get absorbed through your feet. Remember to walk on conductive surfaces, like stone paths, brick walkways, or cement sidewalks. Asphalt and dead wood block electron transfers so find another route for grounding.

Throughout history, our ancestors sought out hallowed ground to heal their wounds, body, and soul. Roman legions even went out of their way to find sacred soil to walk upon, making their way to churches and burial sites blessed by the heavens.

You can find sacred ground all over the Earth: from sandy beaches to grassy backyards, from mountain slopes to desert floors, from wilderness parks and park-like gardens to salty seas and fresh waterways naturally flowing with good things for your body.

12

TAKE YOUR RECOVERY
WORKOUT OUTDOORS

As more and more of us are turning to natural alternatives for healthy living, we are looking outside of the box for our exercise needs; we're taking up walking, running, swimming, and other no-contact activities where fresh air prevails. Think of it as the treadmill versus the terrain trend. Taking your exercise outside not only works your muscles and ligaments while improving your balance, it also helps you avoid the potential EMFs from wireless technologies that are standard inside gyms today. And, on a high note, you'll be increasing those feel-good endorphins that exercise promises.

Mounting studies show that spending time outside is good for our mental and physical health and may be particularly good for our well-being in times of increased stress and anxiety. These studies have linked spending time outside to better health outcomes such as decreases in incidences of diabetes and cardio-vascular mortality, lower blood pressure and heart rate, and better immune system function. In fact, these positive effects are so well-documented that more and more doctors are issuing "nature prescriptions" to help treat a range of conditions from heart disease, hypertension, and diabetes, to chronic stress, depression, anxiety, insomnia, and even PTSD.

"From the report out of the UK defining a 'dosage' of nature (120 minutes) for the first time to the study that calculated the economic impact of protected areas like national parks on peoples' mental health at $6 trillion per year, numerous efforts around the world are underway to advance and promote the health benefits of time spent outside," says Christian Beckwith, executive director of the SHIFT Summit, which works to bring these mounting initiatives to increase people's access to nature for health benefits together for collaboration.[1] Studies show that even just twenty minutes per day spent in nature can lower stress hormone levels, boost self-esteem, and improve mood.[2]

Keith Tidball, PhD, author of *Greening in the Red Zone*, believes part of the reason that going outside is such a good fit for the current situation is because connection to nature fulfills a deep evolutionary need.

"We spent thousands and thousands of years among the rest of nature, that's how we were designed," he says. "It's only in the last couple hundred years that we've become separate from it. But we're compelled to affiliate with nature, which comes to the fore with urgency in times of crisis, because we associate nature with the healing aspects of hope and optimism."[3]

Part of a naturally healthy lifestyle, exercise not only helps you look good, it makes just about every part of your body feel good, too. Shedding those unwanted pounds and keeping them off is one of the most coveted perks of staying active. But exercise also reduces your risk of heart disease, helps manage your blood sugar and insulin levels, works to strengthen your bones and muscles, improves your mood—and your sex life—and promises more restful sleep. In fact, it's just what the doctors order to help reduce your risk of chronic illness and disease and enhance your chances of living longer. Take your exercise outside and, when you add grounding to the mix, the benefits—body and mind along with improving your blood flow and delivering the Earth's electrons where they need to go—get even better.

That's what Marissa Brun does, working nature into her personal workouts, no matter how intense, while advocating the same outdoor setting for her clients. An avid runner, hiker, and yoga enthusiast, Marissa is a licensed psychotherapist, LFMT, and certified ecotherapist with a master's in Clinical Psychology. She works and plays from a nature-based perspective, approaching healing holistically and using mindfulness and ecotherapy frameworks to prioritize the mind/body connection.

She's also a grounding guru, getting behind the science and studies with the knowledgeable air of a professional who both practices and prescribes it. She meets with many of her clients on a trail, at a park, or in an open space, and from there, they will either walk and talk or find a sit spot in nature to deepen the therapeutic experience.

"I believe that our connection to nature greatly impacts our overall wellness and makes us more resilient. Nature-based work is experiential and healing. It allows you to access all of your senses, calm your nervous system, and give your body the nurturing it needs. For many people, nature is a refuge and a place where they can access peace and comfort. Nature aids healing due to its patterns of balance and harmony, which we can tap into anytime we are outside," she explains on her website, *WildSenseTherapy.com*.

After a long, often grueling run, Marissa sits on the ground, explaining that it's necessary to come back to a still place to be present and let your muscles and body heal. In doing so she says you can literally feel the tension and overexertion melt away. Marissa lives and works in Colorado where she is fortunate to be able to immerse in some of the most beautiful wilderness scenery on Earth. That includes her habit of soaking her feet in an icy mountain stream after her hikes and runs, saying that it is a huge part of her exercise recovery program. The grounding properties of water are well documented in their ability to heal cuts and skin ailments, reduce inflammation, and restore energy. "I can't say enough about diving into a lake, pond, or the ocean to recharge and revitalize body, mind, and soul."

Brun also practices yoga outside whenever she can, whether as a daily practice or as part of her exercise recovery program, breathing in the fresh air, stretching, and releasing natural endorphins, the feel-good hormone. She adds that an easy yoga practice also promotes blood flow to help repair your broken-down muscle tissues.

As she tells her clients, grounding helps enhance the benefits of every activity you do outside. To brighten your mood while working your muscles, head outside for some fresh air. The journal *BMC Public Health* found that studies on the topic suggest nature may reduce rumination, putting a stop to those repetitive negative thoughts that keep running through your head and supporting your mental health.[4]

"Being in nature can actually have a similar effect to anti-depressants (without the side effects) as it promotes a healthy balance within our brain while reducing fear, anger, and the production of our stress hormones. Many people (including myself) find a sense of peace, joy, and inspiration from spending time in the outdoors and have seen an increase in confidence by participating in outdoor activities. Our immune systems are positively impacted, and nature has even been shown to reduce blood pressure, muscle tension, and heart rate! Pretty amazing what the wilderness can do for us," she said.

When we exercise in natural environments, we don't feel as though we're pushing ourselves as much, so we work out harder than we would do in a gym, our blood pressure returns to normal much faster, levels of stress hormones such as cortisol and adrenaline drop right back to normal levels, our immune systems improve and it gives us a good mood boost, among many other benefits.

Want to stabilize your blood sugar? Take a stroll around the block after you eat dinner. A study published in the journal *Diabetologia* in 2016 found that just a ten-minute walk after eating helped people with Type 2 diabetes lower their blood sugar levels.[5]

Want to stress less and stay stronger longer? Put regular walks on your schedule. You'll feel a sense of accomplishment by burning calories and banishing cravings—a study published in the journal *Appetite* found that a fifteen-minute brisk walk helped curb chocolate cravings—and lowering your blood pressure, all while strengthening your bones and your stamina.

Studies show that exercise recovery is also more beneficial when taken outdoors. Both passive and active recovery workouts can be good for your body, helping you recover faster after a difficult workout. They also help reduce lactic acid buildup in muscles, eliminate toxins, keep muscles flexible, reduce soreness, increase blood flow, and help you stay fit for your regular exercise routine.

During passive recovery, the body stays completely at rest. It may involve sitting or inactivity, which is further enhanced if you sit on the grass, lean against a tree and read, or rest outside as you wish and let nature do the healing. Passive recovery is important and beneficial if you're injured or in pain. You may also need passive recovery if you're very tired, either mentally or physically, after exercising.

If you're only generally sore, active recovery is considered a better option. An active recovery workout involves performing low-intensity exercise, like walking, yoga, and swimming, following a strenuous workout. It can keep blood flowing and help muscles recover and rebuild. Practicing Tai Chi or yoga can be beneficial for active recovery, especially in the great outdoors. Both help stretch sore muscles and increase flexibility while reducing stress and inflammation.

Rest and recovery are crucial parts of any exercise program. Moderate to strenuous exercise causes muscle fiber damage, small tears in the muscle, and the body healing these muscle tears is how muscles become stronger. The inflammation caused by muscle damage is why muscles are sore is after we use them; good workouts are designed to cause enough muscle damage to create soreness and future strength while not causing so much damage that we become injured. Put simply—the muscles tear and the healing of the muscle creates more strength. Having a speedier recovery does not just assist serious athletes, each of us may be able to do a good workout with a faster recovery. Think about when you exercise and how you handle muscle soreness now. Do you take an Epsom salts bath, ice the muscles, go for a massage, or take an anti-inflammatory? Interestingly, grounding has been studied for faster recovery of the muscles after exercise more than most other areas of research.

After putting your body through a significant amount of stress during a grueling workout, you have to give it time to recover, repair, and ultimately, come back stronger. Elite athletes are known for having specific recovery rituals and routines that they swear by. We reached out to a handful of different athletes and coaches to see what their go-to rest and recovery routines are and weren't surprised to learn that grounding figured prominently in the mix.

Football players are some of the world's toughest athletes, but a severe cramp can still knock them off their feet and out of the game. Several athletes have had severe muscle cramping issues—to the point where they had to leave the game for trainer assistance. Which makes us wonder if the players we see falling on the ground on TV are playing on synthetic astroturf and not on real grass? Think about it the next time you watch a pro game on TV. While they play on FieldTurf at Lumen Field, we have read that the Seattle Seahawks incorporate grounding in workout routines by walking barefoot on their grass football field at the end of practice, which we know helps stop cramping.

In a newspaper article published by the *Pittsburgh Post Gazette*, on September 29, 2021, it was noted that Pittsburgh Pirates utility man Michael Chavis will often stroll out to left field with a yoga mat in hand, go through a routine, and then meditate and perform breathing exercises before his baseball games. He was also grounding in his bare feet long before the health studies about grounding came out. When he saw former Red Sox player Adam Ottavino doing it before a game, he asked him about it.

"I thought that I was the one who invented it, but it's actually a thing," Chavis was quoted to say in the article. "I'm not the only one to do it. Without having any information initially about its health effects, I always felt physically feel better when I did it. So then when I started reading about how continuing to do it can take away inflammation, it just kind of verified and made sense why I felt the way that I did after doing it."

Long-time cyclist Tassana Landy is also a rower. For her, a hard workout on the water is a twenty-plus-mile, four-hour-long row. Her recovery includes a quick nap and a leisurely walk with her dog on wooded trails.

Aika Yoshida is an adaptive climber. For her, a hard workout includes carrying most of her rock-climbing gear, plus food and water, in her pack to the climbing area, using two hiking sticks and a leg brace made out of carbon fiber. Then she climbs six to eight routes, which are about seventy to eighty feet each. After that workout, Yoshida enjoys mobility workouts like outdoor yoga to help her stay loose and keep her pain under control.

The man in charge of recovery for Olympic hopefuls, Ralph Reiff, recommends getting in a lake after running to cool body heat and refresh muscles. In fact, a study in the *International Journal of Sports Medicine* found that athletes who take to the waters for a moderate workout on a recovery day were able to subsequently work out longer than those who took it easy.[6]

In an article in *Scribd*, published on October 22, 2021, Hannan Caldas, a coach with CrossFit Anywhere in Folsom, CA, and a former member of the Portuguese national swim team, explains "Swimming can help start that active recovery process. You're flushing out some of the lactic acid while helping your muscle fibers recover."

Exercising in water is low impact and provides active stretching in every direction. And the faster you move, the harder you'll work. Hydrostatic pressure also circulates blood flow back to the heart, keeping your heart rate ten to fifteen beats lower per minute than on land. And if you are swimming in the salty Mediterranean Sea in one of the world's Blue Zones, like Step does in Greece, you are grounding in a mineral-rich medium that enhances the healing and perhaps promotes longevity.

"There's something special—almost spiritual, even—about touching the Earth. Let's say you've had a challenging day at work. You come home. What's the first thing you do? Take off your shoes, right? When you are barefoot outdoors, something special happens. You feel the ground and suddenly all your anxiety dissipates," say Michael Sandler and Jessica Lee, coauthors of the 2013 book, *Barefoot Running*.

Cristopher McDougall, author of the bestselling book *Born to Run*, wrote about a tribe of super athletes called the Tarahumara who reportedly ran hundreds of miles every day without injury in bare feet or simple leather sandals. He concluded that simple changes in footwear could turn running "from a painful torture into a euphoric human experience."

Runner Ted McDonald, also featured in *Born to Run*, was one of the original runners in the first Copper Canyon Ultramarathon. He discovered the benefits of going barefoot after purchasing "the thickest, most supportive (and most expensive) running shoes he could find. When they only made his pain worsen, he pulled them off and walked back to his house barefoot. That's when he realized that without shoes, his pain went away."

Former Marine Mick Dodge, star of the National Geographic Channel series, *The Legend of Mick Dodge*, is an extreme fitness enthusiast who started "Earthgym" with a partner in the rainforest of Olympic Peninsula in western Washington State. Having lived without footwear since 1991 as a result of painful foot conditions, his extreme exercise techniques include running barefoot upstream in the Sol Duc River.

Before he moved back to the rainforest, in an interview with *Higher Perspectives*, he explained that his feet hurt so bad he "could barely walk. I had always used my walk and run to handle the stress of modern living. So I went home to heal my feet."

"The results came quickly. Not only were my feet healing, but my back pain, neck pain and most of all my heart pain disappeared, and in no time at all I was back into a dead run, stepping out of the sedentary, stressed, sedated and secured living of the modern world. I was dancing as the fire, running as the wind, strengthening as the stone and flowing as the water within, by the simple act of touching with my bare soles and allowing the Earth to teach."

Medical experts say walking is one of the best forms of active recovery. If you're a runner, you can also go for a slow jog. Walking or jogging at a leisurely pace can enhance blood flow and help with recovery. Even a few minutes of movement the day after a tough workout is enough to promote circulation and help reduce stiffness and soreness.

Backing up a slew of studies about the health benefits of walking, a 2018 study of over 50,000 people published in the *British Journal of Sports Medicine* found that regular, brisk walking was associated with a 20-percent reduction across all causes of death.[7] Walking outside in the natural light also helps us sleep better because it triggers a cascade of hormones that help to maintain a balanced circadian rhythm, the body's natural clock.

Why is that important? Because sleep also tops the list of exercise recovery.

When we sleep, our bodies produce growth hormones and synthesize proteins that are used to repair and create new cells. This means that as we sleep, our muscles are growing. Sleep is crucial for repairing muscles that have had a tough workout, but it's also essential for restoring our energy and ensuring that we are rested and alert for the next workout! If you sleep grounded, the effects are even more restorative.

Who knew that exercise recovery could be as simple as a walk in the park and a good night's sleep?

13

EARTH'S SIMPLE CURES

Awareness is curative. That's especially true when it comes to your health, and it has become a mantra of sorts for integrative and traditional health professionals who seek to partner with their patients rather than simply prescribe a pill to cure their ills. We've talked about how the pharmaceutical companies position paid studies to promote their drugs, often manipulating the data to ensure their desired end results. Money is frequently behind their motives as the numbers attest. In 2020, the global pharmaceutical industry realized revenues of some 1.27 trillion U.S. dollars worldwide with consumer spending continuing to grow at an unprecedented rate.[1] COVID-19 certainly affected the pharmaceutical market, raising global drug spending by $88 billion according to a report by the Life Sciences Analytical Institute, and it is projected to add $157 billion to the market within the next few years alone.[2]

The reason behind this points to both doctors and patients who seek relief from a growing number of illnesses that plague their lives. Many of these ailments are a result of lifestyle choices and environmental hazards that can be addressed and alleviated by looking down at our feet and reconnecting with the Earth that gives all livings things just what they need for a healthy, happier life.

As grounding enthusiasts, we've long believed that the body is healthier when we have more physical contact with the natural energetic field of Earth. Scientists have been studying this revelation only in the last few decades, but this health resource dates back to prehistoric ages. Since the dawn of time, humans walked barefoot or wore leather skins on their feet and slept on the ground, oblivious to the energetic activity underfoot that research now shows helps regulate the body's intricate mechanisms. Healers instinctively knew about the natural healing endowment of the Earth, finding cures and connections growing in the soil, thriving in the seas and sands, and flowing abundantly in rivers, streams, and lakes that nurtured body and soul.

As modern-day luxuries and lifestyles insulated us from nature in the past century, many disconnected us from an energy source that's vital to our well-being and were overlooked as causes of the steep rise in chronic diseases, fatigue, and stress that so many of us struggle with today. That energy source is still there though, lying in wait for our footsteps to return to its nourishment.

It's amazing to think that everything in nature was created with our best interests in mind. Nature provides food, shelter, and nourishment, along with the restorative medicine we need, if only we know where to look.

Take our feet, for example. Ingeniously created to carry us wherever we want to go, the foot is designed to make contact with the Earth at the precise anatomical point that triggers healing. Whenever we walk outside on the lawn, the beach, a forested path, and other natural surfaces in our bare feet or leather-clad soles, we automatically invite an electron transfer that keeps our bodies in balance as nature intended. We have discussed the electric fields of our bodies and Earth in great detail, but to make our point here, we want to break down this energy flow in simpler terms.

The Earth harbors a limitless supply of electrons that are constantly replenished by lightning strikes and solar radiation. When allowed to flow into our bodies, these electrons work like antioxidants, disarming the free radicals that make us sick or age. These electrons move through our body via healing channels called meridians, which are stimulated by pressure points located at various places on the body, including the K1 point on the foot. When you walk, you naturally press down on this KI point, activating the meridian that runs up your leg, through the body, and transfers energy via the spinal cord to the pineal gland of the brain. In other words, we are not only taking in grounded energy through our feet, but also the energetic transfer of this health-promoting energy is going directly into the framework of our brain.

All living beings, from parasites to pets and people, are bioelectric life-forms in constant interaction with the environment. Collectively, the cells that make up our bodies form a living matrix through which the body conducts electrical impulses. Cells resonate to particular frequencies and continually transmit and receive energy. Our heart beats to electrical frequencies. Our muscular, nervous, and immune systems also involve electrical currents, and electric fields regulate the movement of nutrients and water into our cells. The natural energy found in the Earth supports the entire electrical cellular framework of our body. Grounding is one of the best steps you can take in terms of your health as you tune into the natural vibrations your body needs to thrive.

There are other Earthly riches that affect your health; among them are the foods you eat and the herbs and botanicals that offer natural, holistically healthy medicinal benefits. Learning about natural sources of nutrition, from vitamins and supplements to wholesome foods, from what to eat and what not to eat not only makes a huge difference in how you feel, but also it can make all the difference in your long-term health.

It goes without saying that Dr. Sinatra is a big fan of natural healing, something he didn't learn in medical school.

As he tells aspiring medical students, "Your patients will be your best teachers, not your professors, who will give you the basics. Listen to your patients because the more alternative treatments you can offer them, the more you will be a resource to them. Some of these patients will come up with amazing discoveries that you never heard of, for example. They will come in and say, 'Hey doc, I started taking licorice root and it's amazing. It really helped me.' Or they will come in with this herb or that herb. You may not know anything about it. What I used to say to my patients over the years is, 'Can you bring me an article on it,' or, 'Tell me where you learned about it, because when patients get better, I want to make sure I share it with others.' My patients provide vital information that I was previously unaware of, making me a more effective healer."

With what we've learned in the last ten years, we have recognized the wisdom of our own bodies. The body wants to heal itself no matter what we do. And what our bodies may lack can, more times than not, be found in nature.

"In addition to learning the benefits of grounding and energy medicine, the public needs to be educated about healthy eating. It's the most important thing you can do for your body. The more people are aware of what they can do to improve and maintain their health, the more they become directly involved in their own self-care. Once they are motivated, they are going to see changes. They'll start to feel better. They might lose some weight. They'll sleep better. Their blood pressure will go down. That's going to give them even more motivation to keep going. Most good doctors become good health coaches. They do a dance with their patients. When doctors can get their patients on the right road and try to educate them in diet and supplements and Earthing and grounding and detoxification measures, whatever it may happen to be, these patients read about things and they bring their doctors material they have researched, and they experiment on their own bodies."

"Years ago, when I first learned about Coenzyme Q10," Dr. Sinatra added, "I prescribed it for a heart patient of mine who presented with a postpartum cardiomyopathy, a very rare and deadly condition that I have only seen twice in my lifetime. As the baby is growing in the womb, it selectively drains energy from the mother's body. After delivery, many new mothers naturally feel fatigue and sometimes depression. But with postpartum cardiomyopathy, because the mother's body has been deprived of vital nutrients, these symptoms become overwhelming which can lead to heart failure. My patient presented with pulmonary congestion and was in obvious heart failure. She had gone from doctor to doctor before she came to see me, and had been advised to get a heart transplant, in addition to the state-of-the-art medicines that other doctors had prescribed for her. She was only twenty-nine years old, and the mother of a two-year-old child and a newborn who was just a few weeks old.

"I decided to put her on Coenzyme Q10, only 10 milligrams three times a day. Like D Ribose and carnitine that power your cells, Coenzyme Q10 (CoQ10) is an antioxidant that your body produces naturally. Your cells use CoQ10 for growth and maintenance. After the first week, she was able to sleep through the night without coughing. After doubling her dose, a week later she was able to walk across the room. Doubling her dose again, after a little more than three weeks, she came into my office and told me she felt almost normal. The hospital found a heart for her three or four months later and wanted to schedule her transplant. Before she made her decision, she called me and said, 'I feel fine. Do I really need this heart?' I answered that it was her decision to make. Fortunately, she made the right choice and refused the heart transplantation and now she's in her mid seventies. That was the first incredible case I ever saw with a COQ10 reversal of cardiomyopathy, a very rare circumstance that more often than not is fatal."

Coenzyme Q10 and grounding share something in common. They're both profound electron donors. And whenever you bring electrons to the table, it's like swallowing a handful of antioxidants. Basically, whenever you bring grounding to the table, you're lowering the pro-inflammatory state because instead of taking handfuls of antioxidants, now you're getting it through the K1 point of your feet, so to speak.

We think grounding is one of the healthiest things we can possibly do to create incredible homeostasis and rid the body of intense inflammation that we all have in this 21st century. The beauty of grounding is that it is free. One of the reasons the Sinatras moved to Florida is that they wanted to be on a seashore. "Because when you walk on the incoming tide at that juncture where the tide comes in and you're walking in water, with your feet in the wet sand, you are really healing the body," Dr. Sinatra explained.

We all know of friends who go on vacations to places like Mexico, Florida, or Southern California, and they come back remarking on how good they feel. What they didn't realize was a lot of them were grounding. They thought they were getting away from their jobs, from cooking, from day-to-day chores, but it was really due to grounding that they felt so much livelier and more in touch with their feelings, their emotions, and their body. The truth is they had less inflammation.

People need to know how they can keep inflammation in check because inflammation is behind the alarming growth in chronic illnesses and pain we see today. Limiting, or better yet, eliminating sugar from your diet is one way to alleviate the harmful effects because sugar fuels inflammation. Reducing processed foods from your diet and eating a heart-healthy diet like the Pan Asian Modified Mediterranean diet is another. Maintaining a healthy weight and getting moderate exercise are key, as is limiting alcohol, which turns to sugar inside your body. Reducing your exposure to pollution including pesticides helps. And it goes without saying that grounding, the simple act of connecting to Mother Earth energy, is a no-brainer to keep inflammation at bay.

Additionally, there are foods you can begin to incorporate into your daily diet that help promote a healthy inflammatory response. Science has shown that fresh ginger can fill this role. Extra virgin olive oil can reverse inflammation in the body as well. Few foods have as many health benefits as green tea because it contains powerful antioxidant flavonoids that help to reduce oxidative stress throughout the body and protect against free radical damage. Plus, green tea contains theobromine, which helps to relax the blood vessel walls to promote better circulation. Pomegranate is one of the richest sources of protective antioxidant flavonoids that support good health. Cocoa powder, and eating dark chocolate—the darker the better—also works.

Securing very pure, clean, healthy food for our families is going to be one of the major challenges of the 21st century and is in our best interests, especially if it fits into the "high vibrational" category.

Medical researchers have long talked about the vibrations of cells, noting the difference between healthy and dysfunctional ones. Illnesses, like cancer and malaria, can slow down and lower the vibration of cells, as can depression and other mental and emotional conditions. Healthy cells pulsate effortlessly. The higher the vibration, the stronger and healthier we become. Lower vibrational energies weaken our vital force and can make us sick. Fear is a lower vibrational emotion; so are rage, jealousy, and grief. On the other hand, love, kindness, joy, and the like are higher vibrational emotions that buoy your spirit and lighten your load.

One of the great things about a high-vibrational lifestyle is that it helps us get back in touch with the natural rhythms of the body and nature. It's about listening to our bodies and emotions, intuitively knowing what's best, and consciously nourishing them with a healthy diet of organically produced, naturally grown food and positive thoughts. It's about grounding wherever and unplugging whenever you can. And it's about making healthy choices and exercising every day so that you can reenergize your body and honor your life.

Follow a Mediterranean-inspired diet, choosing items that are found naturally on Earth. There's something special about the Mediterranean basin that makes people from these places live longer and healthier than almost anywhere else. A lot of it has to do with their grounding lifestyle and nutrient-dense, chemical-free diets that consist of olive oil—the secret sauce of the Mediterranean diet and a proven inflammation fighter— fresh fruit, vegetables, all organic, and wild caught, not farm raised, fish, including sardines, along with a lack of unprocessed, uncontaminated foods, and a little bit of red wine! Organic farmers produce their food products the old-fashioned way, so you should buy from locally sourced, organic vendors when you can. And stay away from synthetically manipulated GMOs and sugar! The 80/20 rule works best here; 80 percent of your diet should come from healthy fats (like olive oils and nuts), colorful vegetables and fruits, and legumes, and just 20 percent from animal protein.

Add seaweed to your diet. It contains a higher concentration of magnesium, iron, and iodine than any other kind of food. Season your food with garlic; it's a natural antibiotic and antiviral remedy that has been used worldwide for centuries. Don't forget to include fresh herbs like rosemary and thyme in your meals—some of the most powerful immune boosters are growing right in your garden!

Sharon Whiteley calls the botanicals of Earth's gardens "essential" for your health. Coming from Mother Earth's abundant medicine chest, they are naturally good for us, made without chemicals or man-made additives that can adversely affect our health. And of course, when you are growing them yourself and putting your hands in the soil, you are grounding.

Take lavender, for example. Records show lavender has been in use for over 2,500 years. The first written record of the healing uses of lavender appears to be that of the Greek military physician Dioscorides in 77 AD who collected medicinal plants from around the Mediterranean Sea. The ancient Egyptians used lavender for mummification and perfume. Romans used lavender oils for cooking, bathing, and scenting the air, and the name is derived from the Latin verb *lavare*, meaning "to wash." The Romans also used lavender oil in soaps and carried it with them throughout the Roman Empire to ward off any number of opportunistic ills.

Before the discovery of antiseptics, lavender oil was used as a cleansing agent to banish bacteria and is still the go-to solution for keeping pests, from scorpions to mice and lice, at bay. Its feel-good fragrance is not a fluke either because its soothing scent invites a restorative sleep that calms the senses. Scientific studies have found lavender oil effective for pain reduction in chronic conditions such as osteoarthritic knees and kidney stones, even successfully testing it to help improve the quality of life for dementia patients. You only need to drizzle a drop or two on a pillow, handkerchief, or favorite fabric, and this gentle elixir eases you into a stress-free state that's at once euphoric and essential.

Essential oils are typically extracted from various parts of plants and then distilled into liquified form, referred to as the essence, for use in what is truly beneficial aromatherapy treatments. These highly concentrated oils are typically inhaled directly or indirectly or applied to the skin through massage, lotions, or bath salts. Inhaling pure, organically grown botanics works by stimulating the smell receptors in the nose, which then send messages through the nervous system to the limbic system—the part of the brain that controls emotions. These are very different from synthetic "fragrances" that have many toxins and chemicals in them. Aromatherapy—a true therapeutic benefit from pure pressed plants—is very different. The word *aromatherapy* has gotten to be very commoditized and is, at times, misunderstood.

Because of their inherent healing benefits, it is no surprise that many organically grown and harvested essential oils are used to manage stress and anxiety, induce calm and comfort, and enhance our well-being. Scientists found that citrusy orange oil has an anxiety-reducing effect on male volunteers who inhaled as few as two to three drops. And pink grapefruit oil has been known to help people control cravings as they diet away excess, unwanted weight gain!

Eucalyptus essential oil is a rock star and has tons of benefits: antibacterial properties for wound care; the ability to improve mental clarity and respiratory conditions; the ability to alleviate pain from headaches and infections; and the ability to relieve congestion, cold, and flu symptoms. Anyone who suffers from headaches and migraines would be well-served to turn to peppermint oil, lavender oil, eucalyptus oil, rosemary oil, and ylang ylang oil.

Tea tree oil's antibacterial, antifungal, and antiviral properties allow it to fight skin infections and conditions and kill off pests like head lice. In addition, it's also a natural hand sanitizer. Other essential oil compounds that can inhibit and fight bacteria and airborn microbes and aid in boosting or helping to protect immunity include sweet orange, rosemary, and even peppermint when diffused into the environment.

Organically grown essential oils can help with inflammatory conditions, too. Rosemary and lemongrass, when applied topically to the skin, can assist in alleviating inflammation and pain. For those moody Mondays and down days, essential oils are a great pick-me-up to elevate your mood and lift your spirits. They include peppermint oil, lemon or lemongrass oil, and rosemary oil.

Lemon essential oil is benefit rich and can help with a wide variety of ailments. It is known for its calming properties and is an antifungal and astringent. Not only does it treat coughs, fatigue, infections, nausea, oral health, and respiratory issues, but it may also be effective at fighting tumors.

Peppermint is invigorating and freshens breath, and it is also good for restoring energy, relaxing muscles, and increasing clarity. It also helps with blood circulation and IBS. Rosemary is also used to combat hair loss; improve memory, liver, and gallbladder function; lower stress; and fight cancer. Overall, it's great for the immune system.

The beauty of botanicals extends to flowers as well. For one thing, plants and flowers oxygenate the air and boost brain cells, which in turn improves memory, clarity, and concentration. Their beauty and fragrance also improve moods, which leads to better health in the long run. Flowers add moisture to the air, too, which helps with dry skin, dry throats, and dry coughs. Studies have shown that having fresh flowers and potted plants around your home or office is linked to an increase in positive energy. The color and scent, specifically, boost energy and creativity, which is something we all could use more of! Not to mention the relaxation they promise when we are arranging them in a vase or a garden outside where we can get grounded as an added health bonus!

Earth's surface is also home to minerals that have proven their mettle in keeping us healthy, such as silver, the world's first true antibiotic. The story of silver dates back thousands of years to an ancient land where artifacts born out of necessity took shape from rocks and minerals colorfully enticing and ultimately useful for everyday living. Picture prehistoric man on the hunt for stones that could stun, slay, and skin their prey some 1.9 million years ago. Sharpening their survival skills, they collected rocks both above, then below, ground, going deep into the dirt to become the first of a long line of miners seeking fortune from the Earth. The more they mined, the more magnificent their finds and the more they were grounding.

The mining of silver is said to have begun between 5,000 and 6,000 years ago in Anatolia, what is now modern-day Turkey, when people dug the first copper mines, serendipitously finding silver alongside the copper veins. Large-scale silver mining had developed in Anatolia by 3,000 BC to meet the demand from the first ancient city states, which used the metal as a common medium of exchange.

Its intrinsic antimicrobial properties were first documented by Hippocrates, the "Father of Medicine," who wrote of using silver to improve wound care and limit infection. Grecians, Romans, and Macedonians were reputed to use silver to keep the immune system strong thanks to its antiseptic properties. Sailors used to throw silver coins into their milk to keep it from spoiling on long journeys before modern refrigeration. This is because silver has oligodynamic properties, which means the metal ions kill living cells and organisms including mold, fungi, viruses, algae, and other microorganisms.

Wealthy families in the Middle Ages, rife with unsanitary living conditions, were known to gift silver spoons, naturally hygienic, to babies to keep bacterial illnesses at bay. English royals were believed to be healthier than the commoners they ruled thanks to their use of disease-defying silver utensils, plates, and goblets.

Hundreds of years later across the pond, silver coins were dropped into drinking water barrels for protection against water-borne illness, and during the Civil War, silver was used to treat syphilis. In the 1880s, the use of silver nitrate in the eyes of newborn infants to prevent post-delivery infections was introduced. First discovered in the 1890s, colloidal silver became many physicians' treatment of choice for boosting the healing process for their patients.

Before the advent of man-made antibiotic drugs in the first half of the 1900s, silver was a leading player in the medical field, where it was commonly used in wound coverings, sutures, and surgical instruments, many still in use today. We even use silver in our modern water purification plants for its enduring sanitizing properties.

It is interesting to note that after Dr. Sinatra's hip replacement, he wore special grounding pajama pants made for him out of silver fabric. Silver is one of the greatest natural conductors for transferring the Earth's energy, while also being a self-sanitizing antimicrobial powerhouse in wound care. Talk about a silver lining! In fact, after just one night of wearing the grounded pants, the swelling on Dr. Sinatra's right leg had gone down. His right leg had been almost twice the size of his left leg after his surgery, but less than two days post-op, the swelling was gone in an amazing accelerated healing. He'll never forget it.

We urge you to step outside and step up your health regimen because nature offers its own medicine. Soak in the sunshine and benefit from a natural dose of vitamin D that plays a fundamental role in maintaining immune system effectiveness and protection against upper respiratory infections, including the common cold, flu, and pneumonia.

Lower your blood pressure and do something good for your heart. Research shows that high blood pressure costs the U.S. approximately $48.6 billion per year and affects one in three Americans.[3] A large June 2016 study found that nearly 10 percent of people with high blood pressure could get their hypertension under control if they spent just thirty minutes or more in a park each week. Unlike the pressures of daily life, nature is undemanding and can elicit feelings of awe that bring a number of health benefits just by being outside.

The benefits of awe are spiritual and physical: regularly experiencing moments of awe has been linked to lower levels of inflammatory compounds in the body. Research has shown that when people walk through a forest, they inhale phytoncides that increase their number of natural killer (NK) cells—a type of white blood cell that supports the immune system and is associated with a lower risk of cancer. NK cells are also thought to have a role in combating infections and autoimmune disorders and in tamping down inflammation, which contributes to a wide range of ailments, including heart disease and diabetes.

A 2015 study published in the *Proceedings of the National Academy of Sciences* found that people who walked for ninety minutes in a natural setting, such as a forest or a nature park, were less likely to ruminate—a hallmark of depression and anxiety—and had lower activity in an area of the brain linked to depression than people who walked in an urban area.[4]

"Accessible natural areas may be vital for mental health in our rapidly urbanizing world," the study authors write. The exact mechanism of how nature helps mood disorders is unclear, but researchers agree that at the very least, time in nature tends to lift spirits—and so much more.

"Never underestimate the spiritual side of natural healing," says Step, who learned about it firsthand when he was studying about the lifestyles of monks. Monks spend a large part of their time meditating and staying mindful as they live out their lives for a higher purpose and seek enlightenment. They respect nature, live simply, and walk barefoot, connecting with the energy of the Earth and the spiritual realm on a daily basis. We can't help but think that the ground, sacred in all respects, and the natural healing you get from grounding, just might be a springboard—or the missing link—for the intuitive awareness, knowing wisdom, and spiritual energy they aspire to.

Optimal health is achieved when body, mind, and spirit are all in synch and is an integral objective in integrative medicine. The ancients knew how important it was to treat the whole person thousands of years ago, so we have a long way to go to catch up. Reconnecting to nature and disconnecting from technology are not only two of the smartest things we can do in terms of our well-being, they are critical to our longevity. When we're spiritually healthy, we feel more connected to not only a higher power, but to those around us. We have more clarity when it comes to making everyday choices, and our actions become more consistent with our beliefs and values. Being more connected to our life purpose and values grounds us into who we are as individuals. Thus, grounding can manifest in a better relationship with ourselves and others around us. Gaining a deeper connection to self leads to increased self-awareness, intuition, and harmony, which enhances how we think and behave.

Slowing down and being mindful are benefits of spiritual wellness. Mindfulness supports us to be more present and focus on the moment. Mindfulness is also a tool to help us be more self-compassionate and better cope with adversities. Our choices in life are more resonant with who we are as individual humans, and when we respond to any situation, we respond with less reactivity and more creativity. It's a way of living according to what motivates us and engages us in life.

Spend time in, and with, nature. Walk around your neighborhood or a nearby park, or go for a hike, as you breathe in the fresh air. Sit on the beach and dip your toes in the water. Get away for a weekend camping trip, and sleep under the stars. Watch the sunset or sunrise, the most calming times of the day. Make time for self-reflection. Reflection allows you to go deeper into yourself and allow the connection with your heart and soul.

Be more forgiving with yourself, and be more focused on the present moment.

Express gratitude and be grateful for all you have, including food, a family, a support system, success, and anything else that stands out. Research has shown that expressing gratitude supports spiritual wellness.

Get outside, take your shoes off, hug a tree, dive into the ocean, plant a garden, play in the sand, and make steps to fully enjoy all the treasures that are found on Earth, and start to heal for free. After all, Mother Nature truly does know best!

CONCLUSION

Increasingly, people of all ages and abilities are turning to natural alternatives for healthy living and are looking outside of the box, literally, for their health needs.

Studies show that even just twenty minutes per day spent in nature can lower stress hormone levels, boost self-esteem, and improve mood.

Experts note that it isn't just our physical health we need to worry about. Our mental health is also suffering from the compounding stressors in our lives. Outdoor exercise provides a mental health boost. Moving outdoors has been shown to reduce anger and depression and improve mood.[1] Exposure to sunlight enhances vitamin D production, which may be partially responsible for this mood-enhancing effect.[2] Research also shows that as little as five minutes of outdoor exercise can improve self-esteem.[3] Any outdoor location will do, but being near greenery or water enhances this effect. Interestingly, low- to moderate-intensity physical activity shows greater improvements in self-esteem than high-intensity outdoor exercise. Activities shown to improve self-esteem include walking and gardening, both of which are key grounding pastimes.

We've given you the whys, whens, and wherefores about grounding in this book, but we also want to give you the opportunity to read a few of Dr. Sinatra's published studies in their entirety, seeing for yourself the critical health benefits of grounding for conditions many of us can help alleviate through grounding: disease-causing ketchup blood and inflammation. To see the studies, please visit *grounded.com.*

IN MEMORIAM

Dr. Stephen T. Sinatra passed away on June 19, 2022, shortly after he finished writing this book.

A cardiologist, educator, and author, Dr. Sinatra was a trailblazer in the field of integrative medicine. An avid interest in energy medicine also led Dr. Sinatra to take part in the discovery of grounding (absorbing the Earth's natural electromagnetic energy) as a complementary healing modality. As you will read in this book, he considered grounding to be one of his most important health discoveries in his exemplary fifty-year career in medicine. He firmly believed that grounding is the greatest free thing you can do for your body, stating that it could help heal millions of people. Empowering people to take charge of their health was Dr. Sinatra's life mission. And it was his wish that this book find its way into the hands of as many people as possible so they could benefit from this abundantly available healing resource. As of his death, he authored more than thirty books and medical textbooks. This book is his last.

ACKNOWLEDGMENTS

There are many people responsible for getting this important book into your hands, from the researchers, scientists, and doctors who worked diligently on studies that confirmed the health benefits of grounding to the people, from the ancients on, who enthusiastically incorporated it into their everyday lives to improve and maintain their good health. To thank them individually would be an impossible undertaking, as their numbers date back millennia and increase with every passing day.

We do want to acknowledge the priceless contributions of our co-author Dr. Sinatra who believed in grounding wholeheartedly and 100 percent. A highly respected, extraordinarily compassionate doctor, mentor, and friend to all, Dr. Sinatra was involved in grounding research from the day he learned about it from Clint Ober. He conducted and personally participated in studies. He informed, educated, and encouraged his patients, colleagues, and communities of health seekers to get grounded, whenever and wherever they could. And he put his medical reputation on the line as he unequivocally declared grounding to be one of the most important health discoveries of his accomplished fifty-year medical career.

Steve passed away shortly after we completed this book. He probably would have balked at the accolades we are including here, but we could go on and on. What we do know is that he would have been thrilled that you strongly consider adding grounding to your daily health regimen. That would be an honor he would not only enjoy, but one he would proudly champion with you.

Thank you for reading this book. Dr. Sinatra often talked about how critical it was to take charge of your own health and implement positive changes that improve your life.

Take the first step and do as the ancients did so long ago and what many of us enthusiastically do today. Reconnect with the Earth. And feel better because of it.

—SHARON WHITELEY

—STEP SINATRA

NOTES

Chapter 2

1 *Advances in Gerontology*, November 5, 2014, 4(4): 283–289.
2 *Hippocrates J Med Ethics Hist Med*. 2014; 7: 6. *Health care practices in ancient Greece: The Hippocratic Ideal*, Christos F. Kleisiaris, Chrisanthos Sfakianakis, and Ioanna V. Papathanasiou.
3 *Boston Globe*, July 5, 2021, by Stan Grossfield.
4 "The Yellow Emperor's Classic of Internal Medicine," *BMJ*. April 5, 2008; 336(7647): 777.
5 Phillip Beach, "Decoding the Chinese Meridial Map," *Muscles and Meridians*, 2010, 153–185, *sciencedirect.com*.

Chapter 3

1 Maurice Ghaly and Dale Teplitz, "The Biologic Effects of Grounding the Human Body During Sleep as Measured by Cortisol Levels and Subjective Reporting of Sleep, Pain, and Stress," *Journal of Alternative and Complementary Medicine* 10(5): 767–76, November 2004.
2 *CDC 2022 National Diabetes Statistics Report*, Jan 26, 2022, Article National Diabetes Prevention Program.
3 Karol Sokal and Pawel Sokal, "Earthing the Human Body Influences Physiologic Processes," *Journal Alternative Complementary Medicine*, April, 2011, 17(4): 301–8.
4 Etymology, origin and meaning of electric, *etymonline.com*.

5   Wilfried Zimmermann, "The Impact of Electricity on Earth, Man, Civilisation, and Culture," The Karl König Institute, *www.karlkoeniginstitute.org*.

6   Gaétan Chevalier, Stephen T. Sinatra, James L. Oschman, Karol Sokal, and Pawel Sokal, "Earthing: Health Implications of Reconnecting the Human Body to the Earth's Surface Electrons," a research study sponsored by EarthFX.Inc. *Journal of Environmental and Public Health*, January 12, 2012.

7   Igor Gorpinchenko, Oleg Nikitin, Oleg Banyra, and Alexander Shulyak, "The Influence of Direct Mobile Phone Radiation on Sperm Quality," *Central European Journal of Urology*, 2014, 67(1): 65–71.

Chapter 5

1   International Commission on Non-Ionizing Radiation Protection (ICNIRP). Statement on the "Guidelines for Limiting Exposure to Time-Varying Electric, Magnetic, and Electromagnetic Fields (up to 300 GHz)," 2009. (2) Institute of Electrical and Electronics Engineers (IEEE). "IEEE Standard for Safety Levels with Respect to Human Exposure to Radio Frequency Electromagnetic Fields, 3 kHz to 300 GHz," IEEE Std C95.1, 2005.

Chapter 6

1   Haider Abdul-Lateef Mousa, MB ChB, MSc, "Prevention and Treatment of COVID-19 Infection by Earthing," University of Basrah, College of Medicine, Iraq.

2   Gaetan Chevalier, "Grounding the Human Body Improves Facial Blood Flow Regulation: Results of a Randomized, Placebo

Controlled Pilot Study," *Journal of Cosmetics, Dermatological Sciences and Applications,* January 2014.

3 M., Eckhoff Connor, "Physiological Testing of Pluggz™ Shoes," *Journal of Inflammation Research,* 2015; 8: 83–96, published online March 24, 2015.

4 Original study commissioned by Sharon Whitely for Pluggz.

5 James L Oschman, Gaétan Chevalier, and Richard Brown, "The Effects of Grounding (Earthing) on Inflammation, the Immune Response, Wound Healing, and Prevention and Treatment of Chronic Inflammatory and Autoimmune Diseases," a research study sponsored by EarthFX.Inc., *Journal of Inflammation Research,* March 2015, PMID 25848315.

6 Rohit Passi, Kim K Doheny, Yuri Gordin, Hans Hinssen, and Charles Palmer, "Electrical Grounding Improves Vagal Tone in Preterm Infants," *Neonatology,* 112, June 2017, Penn State.

7 Passi, et al. "Electrical Grounding Improves Vagal Tone in Preterm Infants."

8 Passi, et al. "Electrical Grounding Improves Vagal Tone in Preterm Infants."

9 Chevalier, G., Mori, K., and Oschman, J. L. (2006), "The Effect of Earthing (Grounding) on Human Physiology," a research study sponsored by EarthFX.Inc., *European Biology and Bioelectromagnetics,* 2, pp. 600–621.

10 Howard K. Elkin, and Angela Winter, "Grounding Patients with Hypertension Improves Blood Pressure: A Case History Series Study, Case Series Abstract, *Alternative Therapies,* Nov/Dec 2018, Vol. 24 No. 6.

11 Haider Abdul-Lateef Mousa, "Prevention and Treatment of COVID-19 Infection by Earthing," University of Basrah, College of Medicine, Iraq.

Chapter 7

1 Agata Blaszcak-Boxe, "Life Science Taller, Fatter, Older: How Humans Have Changed in 100 Years," *Live Science*, July 21, 2014.

2 Angel Lopez-Candales, Paula M. Hernández Burgos, Dagmar F. Hernandez-Suarez, and David Harris, "Linking Chronic Inflammation with Cardiovascular Disease: From Normal Aging to the Metabolic Syndrome," *Journal of Natural Sciences*, April 2017; 3(4): e341.

3 "Bedtime Linked with Heart Health," *European Heart Journal*, European Society of Cardiology, November 8, 2021.

4 Shahram Nikbakhtian, Angus B. Reed, Bernard Dillon Obika, Davide Morelli, Adam C. Cunningham, Mert Aral, David Plans, "Accelerometer-Derived Sleep Onset Timing and Cardiovascular Disease Incidence: A UK Biobank Cohort Study," *European Heart Journal - Digital Health*, Vol. 2, Issue 4, December 2021, pp. 658–666, *https://doi.org/10.1093/ehjdh/ztab088*.

5 Rachel P. Ogilvie, and Sanjay R. Patel, "The Epidemiology of Sleep and Diabetes," *Annals of Epidemiology*.

6 Maurice Ghaly, and Dale Teplitz, "The Biologic Effects of Grounding the Human Body During Sleep as Measured by Cortisol Levels and Subjective Reporting of Sleep, Pain, and Stress," *Journal of Alternative and Complementary Medicine*, October 2004, 10(5): 767–76.

7 Harvard Health Publishing, "How Sleep Deprivation Can Cause Inflammation," Jan. 11, 2022.

Chapter 8

1 Hippocrates. "The oath," *Hippocrates Collected Works*, W.H.S. Jones, (trans-ed.) Cambridge, MA: Harvard University Press.

2 C. Lee Ventola, "Direct-to-Consumer Pharmaceutical Advertising: Therapeutic or Toxic?," v.36(10); National Library of Medicine, October 2011.

3 Joanne Kaufman, "Think: You Are Seeing More Drug Ads on TV? You Are, and Here's Why," *New York Times*, December 24, 2017.

4 Dan Buettner, Sam Skemp, and Beth Frates, "Blue Zones: Lessons From the World's Longest Lived," *American Journal of Lifestyle Medicine*, July 7, 2016.

5 Richard Thompson, "Gardening for Health: A Regular Dose of Gardening," *Clinical Medicine* (London), June 2018; 18(3): 201–205.

6 *healthline.com/nutrition/blue-zones*

Chapter 9

1 Joel Shurkin, "News Feature: Animals that Self-Medicate," *Proceedings of the National Academy of Sciences*, v.111(49), December 9, 2014, PMC4267359.

2 Lindsey Konkel, "Pets Share Owners' Diseases," *Environmental Health News*, September 25, 2012.

3 Arthritis Data and Statistics, National Statistics, Centers for Disease Control and Prevention (CDC), cdc.gov.

4 Stephanie D. Bland, "Canine Osteoarthritis and Treatments: A Review," *Veterinary Science Development*, July 17, 2015.

5 Martin Goldstein, *The Nature of Animal Healing*, New York: Ballantine Books, 2009.

6 Colin Dangaard, "Why Horse Riding Feels So Good: It's All about the 'Earth Spirit,'" *Horsetalk.co.nz*, December 2, 2015.

7 Rodney Habib and Karen Shaw Becke, *The Forever Dog: Surprising New Science to Help Your Canine Companion Live Younger, Healthier, and Longer*, Harper Wave, 2021.

Chapter 10

1 "Tracking SDG 7: The Energy Progress Report," released by the International Energy Agency (IEA) the International Renewable Energy Agency (IRENA), the UN Department of Economic and Social Affairs (UN DESA), the World Bank, and the World Health Organization (WHO). June 7, 2021.

2 Rudolf Steiner, *Illness and Therapy: Spiritual-Scientific Aspects of Healing*, *The Collected Works of Rudolf Steiner*, Forest Row, England: Rudolf Steiner Press, 2013.

3 World Health Organization, "Radiofrequency Radiation and Health—A Hard Nut to Crack (Review)," Lennart Hardell, *International Journal of Oncology*, August 2017, 51(2): 405–413.

4 "High Exposure to Radio Frequency Radiation Associated with Cancer in Male Rat," November 1, 2018, National Institutes of Health.

5 "What You Need to Know about the Cellphone and Cancer Study," Health News, *nbcnews.com*.

6 Cindy L. Russell, "5 G Wireless Telecommunications Expansion: Public Health and Environmental Implications," *Environmental Research*, Aug. 2018; 165: 484–495, *pubmed.ncbi.nlm.nih.gov*.

7 Gaétan Chevalier, Stephen T. Sinatra, James L. Oschman, Karol Sokal, and Pawel Sokal, "Earthing: Health Implications of Reconnecting the Human Body to the Earth's Surface Electrons," a research study sponsored by EarthFX.Inc., *Journal of Environmental and Public Health*, January 12, 2012.

8 Tamir S. Aldad, Geliang Gan, Xiao-Bing Gao, and Hugh S. Taylor, "Fetal Radiofrequency Radiation Exposure From 800–1900 Mhz-Rated Cellular Telephones Affects Neurodevelopment

and Behavior in Mice," *Scientific Reports*, vol. 2, article number: 312 (2012).

9 Jin-Hwa Moon, MD, PhD, "Health Effects of Electromagnetic Fields on Children," *Clinical and Experimental Pediatrics*, 2020.

Chapter 11

1 Modern Institute of Reflexology, Kidney Meridian Chart, *reflexologyinstitute.com*.

2 John Elflein, "Back Pain in the US—Statistics and Facts," Aug. 25, 2021, *statista.com*.

Chapter 12

1 Cassidy Randall, "Why Going Outside is Good for Your Health, Especially Right Now," *Forbes*, April 9, 2020.

2 Randall, "Why Going Outside is Good for Your Health, Especially Right Now."

3 Randall, "Why Going Outside is Good for Your Health, Especially Right Now."

4 "Healthy People with Nature in Mind," Matilda Annerstedt van den Bosch and Michael H. Depledge, BMC *Public Health* volume 15, Article number: 1232, December 11, 2015.

5 Andrew N. Reynolds, Jim I. Mann, Sheila Williams, and Bernard J. Venn, "Advice to Walk After Meals Is More Effective for Lowering Postprandial Glycaemia in Type 2 Diabetes Mellitus Than Advice That Does Not Specify Timing: A Randomized Crossover Study," *Diabetologia* December 2016, 59(12):2572–2578. Epub October 17, 2016.

6 D. Lum, G. Landers, and P. Peeling, "Effects of a Recovery Swim on Subsequent Running Performance," *International Journal of Sports Medicine*, January 2010.

7 Emmanuel Stamatakis, Paul Kelly, Tessa Strain, Elaine M. Murtagh, Ding Ding, and Marie H. Murphy, "Self-Rated Walking Pace and All-Cause, Cardiovascular Disease and Cancer Mortality: Individual Participant Pooled Analysis of 50,225 Walkers from 11 Population British Cohorts," *British Journal of Sports Medicine*, June 2018, 52(12):761–768.

Chapter 13

1 Matej Mikulic, "Global Pharmaceutical Industry—Statistics and Facts," September 10, 2021, *statista.com*.
2 Mikulic, "Global Pharmaceutical Industry—Statistics and Facts."
3 Donglan Zhang, Guijing Wang, and Heesoo Joo, "A Systematic Review of Economic Evidence on Community Hypertension Interventions," *National Library of Medicine*, December 2017; and Alexandra Sifferlin, "The Healing Power of Nature," *Time*, July 14, 2016.
4 Stanford News, "Stanford Researchers Find Mental Health Prescription: Nature," June 30, 2015.

Conclusion

1 J. Barton and J. Pretty, "What Is the Best Dose of Nature and Green Exercise for Improving Mental Health? A Multi-Study Analysis," *Environmental Science and Technology*, 44 (10) (2010), pp. 3947–3955.
2 Dave G. Downing and David C. R. Kerr, "Changing with the Seasons: Does Vitamin D Affect Mood?" School of Psychological Science, Oregon State University, 2014.
3 J. Barton, R. Bragg, C. Wood, and J. Pretty (eds.) *Green Exercise: Linking Nature, Health, and Well-Being*, London and New York: Routledge, 2016, pp. 26–36.

ABOUT THE AUTHORS

Dr. Stephen T. Sinatra was one of the most highly respected and sought-after cardiologists whose integrative approach to treating cardiovascular disease has revitalized patients with even the most advanced forms of illness. He served more than fifty years of clinical practice, research, and study, as chief of cardiology, director of medical education, director of echocardiography, and director of cardiac rehabilitation at Manchester Memorial Hospital in Connecticut. Founder of the New England Heart Center, Dr. Sinatra became known as one of America's top integrative cardiologists by combining conventional medical treatments for heart disease with complementary nutritional, anti-aging, and psychological therapies.

Dr. Sinatra was the bestselling author of more than a dozen books, including *The Great Cholesterol Myth*, *The Sinatra Solution: Metabolic Cardiology*, and *Reversing Heart Disease Now*. Through his books and educating the public on major media outlets including CNN, MSNBC, and *The Dr. Oz Show*, Dr. Sinatra helped tens of thousands of people achieve better heart health and lead long, healthy and active lives.

Sharon P. Whiteley, author, award-winning entrepreneur and innovator, is a grounding pioneer, with three business ventures dedicated to the health benefits of the Earth to her credit. Along with founding a host of industry-leading enterprises and co-authoring books on business, women's leadership, and grounding, she was recognized as Entrepreneur of the Year by Ernst and Young, and has been a guest lecturer at leading institutions throughout the country on entrepreneurship, enterprise creation and innovation, retail development and at industry forums on health and wellness. She was among the first to design and manufacture specialized grounding footwear more than a decade ago and continues to develop mainstream consumer products that promote and facilitate the benefits of grounding. A staunch proponent and expert on nature-based healing, she says grounding changed her life, attributing her recovery from chronic bouts of Raynaud's Disease and a sudden heart attack to her daily regimen of reconnecting to the Earth.

Step Sinatra, Wall Street wizard turned healer, says grounding saved his life against all odds. He is a master healer and is the co-founder of *grounded.com*, a site created to get the word out about grounding and healthy lifestyles. A former Wall Street trader, California winemaker whose *freespiritwine.com* featured organic varietal wines, virtual Chi-Gong and meditation teacher, and the spirit-lead travel retreats at *ageless.com* are his brainchild.